The Complete

Reiki

Handbook

Basic Introduction and
Methods of Natural Application
A Complete Guide for Reiki Practice

LOTUS LIGHT
SHANGRI-LA

Reiki is an effective method of healing and for the stimulation of mental and spiritual growth. Nevertheless, it does not mean that a physician, non-medical practitioner or psychotherapist should not be consulted whenever there are any indications of a serious physical disorder.

Careful research has been carried out with the information and exercises presented in this book which I have presented to the best of my knowledge. The author and the publishers will not be liable for any kind of damage resulting directly or indirectly from the application or utilization of information given in the book.

Note: The drawings in this book show naked bodies in order to demonstrate the Reiki hand positions clearly and to convey the feeling of intimacy, freedom and love which is the very essence of Reiki. The pictures are not intended to suggest that Reiki has to be practiced in the nude. Normally Reiki is not performed naked, and participants of all Reiki seminars also remain fully clothed.

6th English edition 2000
5th English edition 1999
4th English edition 1997
3rd English edition 1996
2nd English edition 1995
1st English edition 1994
Lotus Light Publications
P.O.Box 325
Twin Lakes, WI 53181
The Shangri-La Series is published in cooperation
with Schneelöwe Verlagsberatung, Federal Republic of Germany
©1990 reserved by Windpferd Verlagsgesellschaft mbH, Aitrang
All rights reserved
Translated by Wilfried Huchzermeyer
Edited by Christopher Baker and Judith Harrison
Cover design by Wolfgang Jünemann, color drawing by Roland Tietsch
Illustrations by Roland Tietsch
Layout by Monika Jünemann

ISBN 0-941524-87-6
Printed in the USA

The Complete Reiki Handbook

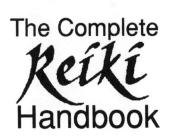

Dedication

For Manu

Acknowledgments

I would like to thank all the many teachers with whom I was fortunate to have direct or indirect contact. I would also like to extend special thanks to my parents, my brother, Matthias Carstens, Horst Kosche, Renate Lorke, Wolfgang Grabowski, Roland Geßler, Hans-Jürgen Regge, Vera Suchanke, Brigitte Müller, Phyllis Lei Furumoto, Dr. Mikao Usui, Dr. Chujiro Hayashi, Hawayo Takata, Manuela Lübeck, Cinderella, Bagheera and to the greatest of all teachers, Life, which God gave to me.

From the very beginning, my greatest concern in writing this book has been to inspire others to accept full responsibility for their own lives. The more each of us infuses our own life with love, truth and knowledge by this greater acceptance of self-responsibility, the speedier the process of transformation toward the "New Age" will be—and God will be at home on the earth once more.

Table of Contents

Preface

We owe very special thanks to the author of this book, as he describes in a clear concise fashion a method of treatment which—irrespective of all challenges, obstacles or legal restrictions—offers therapeutic possibilities to biological medicine that point to even greater future possibilities in the face of the challenges confronting naturopathy and empirical medicine today.

Reiki treatment eludes all measurable criteria and is beyond scientific explanation. It deals with energies and forces which are not immediately intelligible to us "enlightened", modern human beings, living as we do in the computer age. To understand Reiki, we require a view of life which does not exclude many unknown phenomena (some of which are only accessible to us through esoteric knowledge) in the microcosm and the macrocosm as actually existing alongside scientifically ascertained data.

Every human being has the innate capacity to work with Reiki. Those who have an open-minded attitude toward life and to the wonders of nature that surround them know that there are a host of inexplicable, incomprehensible influences affecting their feelings, behavior and also their bodies, their very well-being as well as their illnesses. However, to apply Reiki practically for yourself or others, channels must be opened in certain regions of the various bodies (both physical and subtle). This opening process is performed as an initiation by a Reiki master trained in the traditional way.

As is the case with any other therapeutic application, Reiki may cause "side effects" resulting from cleansing processes which may occur. Therefore, we recommend gaining sound knowledge of the method itself and its forms of application as given by Reiki masters at training seminars. This book will help to broaden the knowledge thus gained and provide more insight into Reiki so that it may be applied with greater ease and care. In view of further limitations of biological medicine likely to manifest in the future, Reiki will gain in importance, especially in view of the fact that it does not cause any permanent damage. It is an invaluable aid and an enrichment to alternative medicine.

This book is especially commendable as it establishes connections between Reiki and biological medicine by pointing out combinations possible with herbal extracts, homeopathic preparations, Schüssler salts, and the spagyric remedies which have been rediscovered. The combined action of Reiki energy and natural medicinal substances, some of which have been known from time immemorial, speed up and improve the therapeutic effect to a considerable degree.

May this book be helpful to all those who wish to assist others through the healing process in a responsible manner, and may it inspire all who read of it with knowledge and skill and with even greater respect for the unique creation of each individual. Most of all may it guide you along your own path.

Hanover, April 1990
Horst Kosche, President of the German
Society for Alternative Medicine Inc.

Introduction

I feel there is much you can glean from this book. What you actually gain, however, greatly depends on your own momentary situation in life.

If you have not yet received initiation into the Reiki energies, the "Reiki Handbook" will provide you with a fund of information on the possibilities and limitations of Reiki. I have also included a number of potential applications, many of which can even be applied without the Reiki initiations, such as the practical suggestions in Chapters 9, 10 and 11. If you are interested in any of the various methods of energy healing, the exercises and detailed instructions on chakra work will offer you invaluable pointers.

If you have already been initiated into the Reiki energies by a Reiki master and have received the attunements that go with it, you will find useful information on which you can base your practical work with Reiki in the future. Unfortunately, two seminar days are insufficient to provide full insight into the many potential applications of Reiki, which is very unfortunate, as Reiki is a wonderful starting-point for all journeys and excursions into your own Self. Whether it be healing for yourself or others, single or group meditation, work with precious stones, transformation work for your personal development, aroma therapy, journeys to other energy levels or overcoming karma—all this and much more is possible with Reiki.

This book offers many practical suggestions to help you intensify your contact with Reiki energy, and provides important background information and many stimulating ideas for further exploration; like a faithful companion, may it accompany you on your Reiki journeys into your true Self.

If you apply Reiki energy frequently to make contact with your true Self, for instance, or to open up to a greater capacity for love, you are already on the way of "Reiki-Do" and can follow the "path of healing love". Many people have not yet discovered this simple and effective path of transformation, simply because they know nothing or too little about it. The "Reiki Handbook" should be helpful in closing this rift.

The "Reiki Handbook" will also assist you even if you are already working as a therapist in a healing profession by providing additional pointers to effectively complement your present working methods with Reiki energy.

How to use this book

I have structured this book carefully so that you can use each chapter individually or simply to gain initial information on each field of application of Reiki energy. If however, you intend to use Reiki in therapy or in addition to your therapeutic work, you might consider studying the entire text in greater detail. It is not necessary to follow the given order of chapters, but please keep in mind that some chapters are complementary and should be studied together.

Chapter Twelve is important for professional use as it provides basic information enabling you to adapt your Reiki work to concurrent medication.

If you apply Reiki mainly for use in the home, the chapter on whole body treatment and the therapeutic index in the appendix will be a powerful tool, helping you deal more effectively with your own and your family's minor complaints.

If you want to walk with Reiki along the "path of healing love", it would be best to re-read those passages which especially appeal to you, and to perform those exercises which you enjoy the most. This is the easiest way of staying in touch with Reiki and this is an important factor, as it is decisive for successful Reiki that you make contact with Reiki energy as often as possible. I recommend that you follow the pleasure principle in Reiki and avoid making it a "duty", as Reiki is a life-giving force and healing love, not a strait-jacket.

I hope you enjoy reading this book and that you have a lot of fun experimenting with Reiki!

Chapter One

Reiki-Do:
The Path of Healing Love

Reiki is a Japanese word meaning "Universal Life Energy", the divine life-giving force. "Do" is also Japanese, and has the same meaning as the Chinese term Tao, which is "path" in English. In Japanese the "Do" is affixed to certain terms to indicate that the activity to which they refer can also be a way of life at the same time, helping the student to develop his personality and to attune his life to the rhythms of the universe. Judo, bushido, aikido and kendo are some of the examples best known to us in the West.

Living with Reiki has become this kind of path for me. I gradually became aware of its characteristics which then combined to form a harmonious system, which I call Reiki-Do. Reiki-Do includes, among other things, the traditional Usui-system of Reiki.

The Japanese theologist Dr. Mikao Usui, after whom this system was named, discovered the long-forgotten art of healing by transferring Universal Life Energy after many years of intensive search in the writings of the disciples of Gautama Buddha. This was around the end of the last century while Usui studied in a Buddhist monastery. After a subsequent 21-day period of fasting and meditation, he was given an initiation into this art through universal life forces. From this point of time onwards Dr. Usui possessed the ability to transfer Reiki energy and assist other human beings to become channels of Reiki energy. Reiki was then brought to the Western world through grand masters in direct spiritual succession, namely Dr. Chujiro Hayashi, Hawayo Takata and Phyllis Lei Furumoto. If you wish to read the complete present day story of Reiki you may study it in the books of Baginski and Sharamon or Paula Horan. These authors have given a very sensitive account of it.

The traditional Usui-system of Reiki is the foundation of my Reiki-Do. Its initiations and the symbols and methods connected with them are what makes Reiki-Do possible in the first place. I discovered many explanations and practical applications of Reiki techniques through my experiences with the I Ching, an ancient Chinese oracle, the chakra teachings, and the more inward style of martial arts in Asia. The ancient "Huna"-teachings of Polynesia were also very stimulating for me with regard to Reiki-Do. The most important methods of Reiki-Do are described below in the text.

Before examining them more closely I would like to first give some basic information on the "whys" and the "wherefores" of Reiki-Do. It is not possible, of course, to convey experience to its fullest extent through a book which is why I also hold seminars for practical experience. What this book will do for you, however, is enable you to look things up again and find inspiration for new discoveries.

I personally experience the essence of Reiki as love; an all-embracing divine vibration, emanating joy and life. Many people may have difficulty coming to terms with what would initially appear to be a very abstract standpoint—and admittedly there are no few whose claims to understand all-embracing love are little more than fond illusion. I am not sure whether one's intellect can really understand love and open to it on all levels, but if I open to greater contact with others, Reiki brings me in touch with the truth of love which is beyond reason. Since each person has to proceed along his or her own path to God and thus to Love, my experience has shown that it is important to have many practical options available to be able to find your own path.

One by one I will describe many of the paths I have explored with Reiki and which I have experienced as being meaningful. However, an introduction to the various potentials inherent in Reiki-Do, the "path of healing love", and to my ideas regarding its theoretical background will help you to understand the practical methods which follow more easily. These ideas are my own personal view and naturally color my approach to Reiki. Perhaps you will develop another view which is more relevant for you. I would welcome this, as this is what keeps Reiki-Do alive. Before discussing the practical possibilities of Reiki-Do, however, I will first deal with the actual way Reiki energy works.

Reiki is neither positive nor negative. It is the greatest vibration of life energy available to a human being. This vibration has a divine quality and for this reason does not exclude anything. It allows us to make contact with the impulses alive in the world, thus conveying "oneness". All human problems and physical disorders are ultimately due to the illusion of "separateness" from the world.

Moved by this ensuing feeling of loneliness, people seek partnership and security. Some try to achieve security and love through power. They believe they have to transform the world so that it takes care of their needs. In doing so they always have to guard themselves against others who might otherwise frustrate their efforts and therefore adopt a competitive mentality. This stage of consciousness

14

is very far from any feeling of unity with God. Others believe they first have to expiate their guilt in order to be entitled to God's love and support once more. These people often struggle their whole lives to expiate the supposed guilt. They never succeed, of course, because this guilt is an illusion. Often such people are lucky if they eventually have a certain experience which conveys to them that they are finally free from all such guilt. They are then finally able to perceive the truth of who they are, which has been there waiting for them all along.

The Reiki attunement or a Reiki session may sometimes provide this kind of experience, because during the process a consciousness of unity becomes more perceptible through direct contact with this energy. Some are absolutely convinced that the path to God can be found through avoidance of all enjoyable things. Therefore, they believe they have to outgrow "fun and games", sensuality and sex, food and drink, dance and celebration. But does a human being not approach the status of a machine if he denies and suppresses all pleasure? In this way, does he not move further away from God, who is him/herself the personification of vitality, joy and love?

These "life strategies" are all different manifestations of the same illusion of separateness from the divine. Burdened by these, man believes that in no case may he be allowed to shape his life according to the pleasure principle, and that under no circumstances may he be allowed to be happy. Out of this illusion of guilt, he then misinterprets obstacles in his path as a sign that he should be even harder on himself, placing yet more duties and "have to's" on his shoulders.

What happens now to these strategies when a person receives the Reiki energy, if he really allows it to enter himself?

In the seminars leading to the Reiki First Degree (the introduction into the Usui-system of Reiki) I often observe the same phenomenon; the participants join the course on the first day with a rather sceptical attitude. They usually do not talk much to one another or show their feelings. They behave as if they were isolated from the rest of the world—which indeed most of them are. After the first attunement to Reiki energy however, they begin to talk to each other. They smile a lot more and I observe that people seem to warm up more and more and become livelier with each attunement. At the end of the course they all tend to treat each other as if they had been close friends for a long time. They show their feelings, hug each other, express interest in the lives of others and find their own center, sometimes with tears welling up when a participant becomes aware of his long-standing isolation, which now suddenly gives way to the sensations of love and union and the resultant feelings of happiness and joy. After frequent Reiki treatments a client may have a similar experience, although not as quickly. A Reiki recipient becomes more lively, and opens once more to his or her own loving inner links with the world.

There is a basic rule with Reiki that the recipient of Reiki energy decides for him or herself on the subconscious level whether and how much life energy he or she will take in. Reiki is never sent or forced into the body, but rather it is drawn in by the recipient. Accordingly, Reiki considers, in its effect, the individual needs of each person. Universal Life Energy gives human beings the personal freedom of dissociating themselves, if that is what they want, and it reinforces opening and living growth, if that is their choice.

All living beings carry the same divine energy within themselves which is actually what gives them life. In a certain sense everyone is God, because his or her innermost core is divine. Our freedom of choice itself is an important part of this divinity. To become aware of and know this freedom is an important step in the development of each human being. Acceptance of freedom in shaping your own life also implies acceptance of your own individuality. If I am able to accept myself as I am, I am also automatically confident and upright in my dealings with other people and especially in my contact with God. A free person can face God in open truthfulness. There is no need for him to beg for grace or make himself humble for reasons of false guilt.

Firmly rooted in freedom human beings can treat each other with mutual respect and honor the individuality of others. No one has to play "hide-and-seek" just because he fears he must not show his true face to his fellow man.

From the onset Reiki proceeds on the foundation of mutual respect. In fact Reiki does not allow us any other motivation, as Universal Life Energy does not permit any therapeutic abuse. It may however happen that in the process of Reiki treatment suppressed feelings rise to the surface, sometimes bursting forth unexpectedly in a violent eruption. This may frighten someone who has never experienced this kind of release, but Reiki will not cause harm in any way.

People who use Reiki often quickly raise their own life-force energy. "Fate" then seems to deal them fewer blows by way of accidents and diseases. Reiki also seems to help them grow into their own identity without external pressure. The individual's life-force energy finds increasingly harmonious possibilities of expressing itself, because old blockages are gradually dissolved and new ones cannot be created. Regular contact with Reiki energy enhances creativity and, along with it, the active expression of Self. We are not driven by fear, but rather motivated by joy; the pleasure principle then becomes the inspiration to create. The shackles of compulsion can be discarded more easily and we are then able to enter new, healthier relationships. Naturally, this fundamental restructuring may at first cause insecurity and anxieties and some effort may be required to bring these new experiences into perspective. A new vitality can be felt as Reiki energy infuses your entire life. Until you actually experience this new vitality directly it is hard to imagine that something so simple can create such an entirely new way of being. This is, in essence, the effect Reiki has on our psychological state. Detailed observation shows that it has a very similar effect on our physical organs. The Universal Life Energy relaxes those parts of the body which it is allowed to enter. Tension brings anxiety and hostility into your life; wherever there is love, hostility and tension cease. This is why acute inflammations ease under the effect of Reiki, for they are symptoms of a conflict bound to erupt when you resist life, and blockages occur. Reiki opens other, more harmonious pathways, and in flowing the blockages will be dissolved.

Relaxation is followed by stimulation of the metabolism as a new vitality flows into the organism. All of a sudden the detoxification processes become revitalized and are subsequently capable of eliminating old waste products while preventing the accumulation of new ones. In this way more and more areas of the body are opened to the life-force energy and thus to relaxation.

The more the subtle and organic channels are cleared, the more responsive we become to stimuli in our environment. After having dissolved many blockages which narrow perception we develop a more holistic perception of reality.

As previous energy blockages are released and greater flow becomes possible, increased vitality results.

The function of psychic and physical protective mechanisms such as the immune system, instinctive perceptions, the skin with all its protective functions and the energetic shielding of the aura is improved. There are two prerequisites for achieving all this; firstly the traditional attunement for the opening of Reiki energy and secondly regular treatment.

In my experience some people hesitate to become involved in a Reiki seminar because they have little understanding of its basic principles. It is therefore important that you address everyone individually with the appropriate language which most appeals to his or her innermost heart. Every human being seeks love and its encompassing sense of unity, but each also expresses this basic need in a different way. One person may say he wants to get well again, another would like to get closer to God, and yet another may want to experience samadhi. Since the need is essentially the same, although manifesting in its various forms, the Reiki teacher must have the ability to convey his or her experience in a comprehensible manner so that the message can be understood by people from different walks of life. It is important to understand that Reiki is essentially free of all dogma or rules which makes it accessible for people of all creeds.

We cannot assume that everyone who participates in a Reiki course will subsequently apply Reiki energy on a regular basis. The short period of time during the seminar is also insufficient to show each participant the manifold possibilities inherent to Reiki. Many participants lack the preliminary information needed to subsequently explore Reiki on their own. How can we expect them to do so? Who would think of working on his chakras if he does not even know about them or how they work? Or, to give another example, how is one supposed to know that Reiki can actually cure a house plant of mites?

In esoteric circles one occasionally hears the preconceived notion that a certain level of maturity is required for practicing consciousness expanding methods and that those who do not practice are not "ready" yet. I tend to disagree. In my experience, what is actually lacking is the individual key stimulating curiosity and eagerness to learn.

Today we tend to put too much emphasis on rationalization and logic. Whatever eludes intellectual understanding initially frightens or bores us, because it seems inaccessible. People generally need some external form at the outset for their orientation to break through this block, a form which is intelligible to them and which forms a basis for subsequent developments of their own. It is the same as with the ancient "inner martial arts" of Tai Chi Chuan in which certain motions are practiced at first, in order to make the student acquainted with the basic principles of this art. Later this gives way to greater freedom of personal expression within the framework of the universal laws of motion, the living interaction of yin and yang.

Similarly, everyone who has participated in a Reiki course now has a comparable basis for practise at their disposal in the form of Reiki-Do, the path of healing love.

The System of Reiki-Do

I created the following image in order to illustrate the effects of Reiki. The yin/yang symbol represents the eternal flow of life energy. It is constantly flowing from one pole to the other and, even while flowing, changes its quality in order to create the right conditions for the reversal of the movement. This cosmic rhythm affects the lives of human beings, as represented by the ray of energy emanating from the center of the monad. As soon as this energy enters a living being (center of the alpha omega or lemniscate), it activates processes of growth. The left side of the lemniscate represents the yin pole, the formative, material condition; the right side, the yang pole, the ideal, free condition in the process of life. On the yang side, man is aware of his freedom and his potential. He is full of self-confidence and enters into new situations in life to gain experience and test his abilities. Ideas are born, plans are conceived and the future is mapped out. Then he starts implementing his plans and realizing his projects. Since the resources and space on earth are limited, and since he has not recognized the portion to which he is entitled, he will inevitably clash with other people who likewise wish to realize their own plans. The further he advances, the greater the obstacles become. The frustrations (obstacles to his progress) in the outside world create physical and mental blockages inside him. He falls ill, is weakened and becomes discontent with life. And if he then realizes that all his efforts ultimately will not help him, he will desperately search for a solution to his plight.

Eventually it may dawn on him that "solutions" are not to be found in the outside world. It becomes apparent that the real solutions to life's challenges lie within oneself. The more he becomes involved in recognizing and removing the inner causes of his problems, the more vitality develops. New ideas come to mind and new faculties are developed. Now he has lived through the yin loop of one particular plane of experience and re-enters the yang side—but on a higher level of experience. He has gone through and assimilated many new experiences. All the knowledge derived from them and the new resulting capacities are now at his disposal. If he has to face these or similar experiences once more, he will be able to deal with them with greater authority and proficiency. But this does not happen. The clock cannot be turned back. Already he finds himself once more making plans and developing projects, right in the midst of a new yang loop which will make him face new problems. Soon he will re-enter the outside world to realize his ideas. A new cycle of life begins...

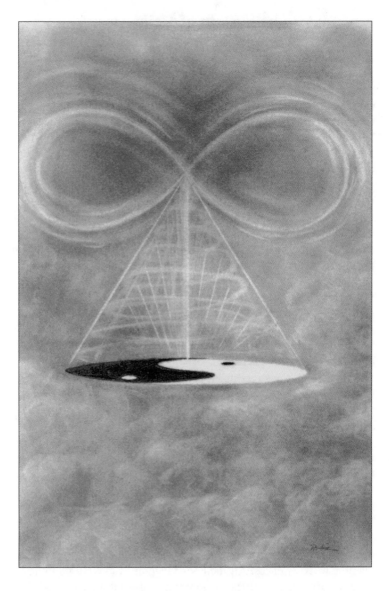

Fig. 1: Life is an interplay of yin and yang

This law of evolution, further development through the confrontation of life with the limited possibilities of inert matter, is basically impossible for us to alter. But we can influence the size of the yin and yang loops. The more conscious, alive and sensitive a person shows himself to be in a learning situation, the more subtle the resistance is which is sufficient to initiate constructive confrontation with the obstacles to life energy. Like an aikido master he anticipates every aggressive impulse of his environment and uses its own movements to move it back into harmony without any major impediments. Massive "incentives" for development such as serious illnesses, accidents or other blows of fate are not required to initiate a process of development. To ensure an easy pace of learning, a person should be as free as possible from blockages which impair his sensitivity and reactions. Through its relaxing effect Reiki creates the best conditions for this.

Reiki-Do basically offers three methods for personal growth which we can realize either individually or as a whole. Our mental and spiritual faculties will determine which of these possibilities should be considered for our first step. These are:

Inner Reiki-Do

Outer Reiki-Do

Synergystic Reiki-Do

The inner Reiki-Do uses Reiki meditation techniques described in Chapter Eleven. They can be supplemented by using precious stones, fragrances, and sounds, i.e. you can use various stimuli to evoke the senses. Here we can already see that inner Reiki-Do is not primarily focused on achieving given goals, but rather follows the pleasure principle. The whole body treatment is its most important method. It is a great pleasure to experience it. Those who are introverted by nature may prefer the deep inner awareness which occurs as a result of self-treatment. Inner Reiki-Do is a mystical path. If we follow it for a long period of time, our awareness will develop and we will feel more alive. If you are interested in finding out more about inner Reiki-Do, you will find valuable suggestions in Chapters 4, 9, 10, 11, and 13.

Outer Reiki-Do is essentially the specific application of Reiki energy. Single or success-minded (i.e. more extroverted) persons generally want to see more immediate results. They can work more specifically on their problems and enjoy results through chakra work with Reiki, the use of precious stones, sounds and fragrances, as well as other supplementary methods for the dissolution of blockages. Contemplation on the rhythms of life, the eternal laws of evolution, as recorded in the I Ching, the ancient Chinese book of oracles and wisdom helps to create awareness of our own potential and to define our current state of affairs, from which we can plan further development. If you are interested in outer Reiki-Do you will find practical suggestions in Chapters 2, 3, 5, 6, 7, 8, 9, 10, 12 and 14.

As the name itself suggests, synergystic Reiki-Do fuses the methods of inner and outer Reiki-Do into a harmonious whole. It is suitable for all those who have already gathered a considerable amount of experience and therefore realized that the pleasure principle and a success-oriented attitude do not necessarily exclude each other, but rather complement each other in a meaningful way. If you are prepared to accept this key insight, you will enjoy this book and sampling all its various suggestions.

The Reiki Principles

Today, as we are on the threshold of a new age, many people find it hard to adjust to the changes inherent in our times. Reiki is a tool which will help people to find it easier to adjust to these changes. My suggestions are meant to awaken your curiosity and to help you generate your own methods of using Reiki energy.

The basic characteristics of Reiki-Do have already been outlined, but its presentation would be incomplete if we omitted to refer to the original Reiki principles as handed down by Dr. Usui. These are taken from the diary of Hawayo Takata. I feel it is important to quote them, as at times there are several variations, and occasionally some Reiki masters have different ones. Perhaps you will find these original principles as helpful as I do. I believe they go well with Reiki. They run as follows (according to Bart Simpson):

Don't get angry—just for today

This rule has always touched off various reactions within me; why shouldn't I be angry? After all, I'm entitled to my own feelings! By George, I won't allow them to be simply outlawed! What's this stupid idea? And there I was, fuming. Could it be that Dr. Usui wanted to use this rule to show just how downright trivial the things usually are that spark our anger? If I cannot agree with this rule I am free to put it aside and not get more upset about it! But that is exactly what I do not do. I get angry about it rather than doing the obvious thing! So I am wasting my time. Oh yes, indeed, just for today don't be angry ...

Do not worry—just for today

I am constantly worrying. I don't know what your trip is and that really worries me. Maybe you're a happy-go-lucky person and you leave all the worries to me! Everybody thinks you're the greatest because you won the personality contest. But me, nobody likes me because I have all these worries, and they're written on every line in my face. Gee, if you would only worry just a little! Then there would be one less person I would have to fear and I wouldn't have to worry because you obviously don't. If just for today I didn't worry, I might actually enjoy my life. But that is too easy. I cannot do that. Then I wouldn't be worrying about the problems of the world, and it would collapse without me!

Honor your parents, teachers and elders
(Be kind to your neighbor)

Actually, are my neighbors kind to me? I don't know about that. And what happens if I am kind to them and they misunderstand me? That would be too embarrassing! I think I'll wait until they are kind to me. Let them take the first step. Maybe I'll be kind next time.

Earn your living honestly
(Earn your daily bread honestly)

But that is what I do, what all of us do! Even my tax return is accurate! Okay, just a little doctored ... But still quite acceptable and perfectly legal. Am I not in the right? Just think of how the state pours our money down the drain. So what does it matter, a few bucks more or less? And it is very rare that I pretend to be sick, and take a few days off rather than work. And what difference does it make anyhow? Those big shots earn enough money as it is. They are the ones who should ask themselves if they earn their daily bread honestly! Folks like us have to scrimp and save just to get our piece of the pie. Those boys at the top are clever with their offshore trusts. My expense account is my slush fund. Who else is going to look after me? So as far as I'm concerned I'm making an honest living.

Show gratitude to every living thing
(Be thankful for your blessings)

What blessings are you talking about anyway? Today it was swelter-
ing outside, yesterday it rained. There's never anything decent on
the TV, so if nothing else comes up I'll have to go to the movies
again. After all, I can't be a couch potato all the time and I can't zone
out on booze either. Hmm! Blessings ... I don't know about that. I'll
ask my girlfriend tomorrow. Maybe she's has some idea. But I should
call her from work, it's cheaper ...

As you can see, the Reiki principles do have a little wisdom. You
may not agree with them like Bart Simpson, but they help to show us
where we stand. They point out our basic attitudes to life and the
hang-ups that we tend to dwell on. They are not commandments in
the biblical sense, but they guide us towards a greater understanding
of ourselves.

The Effects of Reiki on Life Style

Many people lead very hectic, disharmonious lives. Emotional highs
and stressful situations alternate at frequent intervals and are so
marked that the intensity of the experiences themselves place too
great a strain on our nerves and organs. With time these situations, if
repeated often enough, result in apathy, an attitude of resistance and
cynicism. Release is usually sought by pursuing superficial experiences. This search creates even more stress because no lasting con-
tentment or harmony is found in these experiences. Thus life is run
either by our craving for outside stimuli, or by our resistance to truly
experiencing them. Whatever we experience only satisfies us tem-
porarily and for the most part cannot be integrated into our deeper
nature, because it has little to do with the real lessons we are here to
learn during this incarnation.

Reiki reduces the extreme highs and lows of life if it is applied
regularly. Gradually a life style is developed which is balanced inwardly as well as outwardly. By becoming more in tune with your
inner Self, stress and the feeling of being out of touch simply disappear. The quality of your life improves as you more easily integrate
the experiences which cross your path. A sense of peace arises as
you realize that the lessons you have learned enrich your personality. Physical and mental afflictions improve and often disappear or

are suddenly cured by medical means which so far may have been ineffective without the boost Reiki provides. Reiki supplies a continuous flow of energy which causes the Third Eye, which is responsible for the recognition and realization of the ideal path for each of us, and the energy center, the root chakra, to work together in harmony.

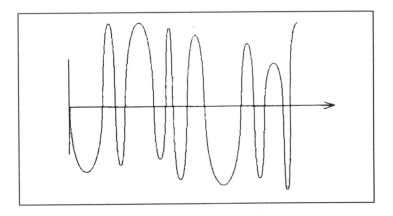

Fig. 2:
Above: stressful life; bottom: stress release with Reiki

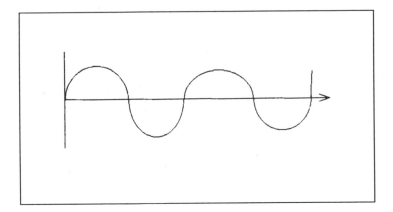

Chapter Two

Possibilities and Limitations of Reiki Application

Reiki energy basically has five effects:
It brings about deep relaxation
Dissolves energy blockages
Detoxifies
Supplies healing universal life-force energy
Increases the vibrational frequency of the body

All these processes constantly interact. Through deep relaxation and its "letting go", tension (blockages) on the physical and mental-emotional plane are dissolved. Release of tension and blockages then permits a normal flow of life energy in all areas and a more rapid removal of waste products and toxins. Once the organism has been thoroughly detoxified it has more scope for its vital processes and can therefore receive, store and use more life energy. The more life energy there is in the body, the higher its frequency becomes, and through it we come in contact with the Universal Spirit (Christ, Universal Mind, or the Goddess). This contact, with all-embracing unity (love) creates faith (trust in universal life-force energy). A human being now knows that the universe is there to support him, accepting him unconditionally. The resultant feeling of security brings about a state of deep relaxation which grants access to levels of experience that were previously inaccessible. However, if you overextend these new-found faculties you may again cut yourself off from divine Love. Tension sets in, and a new cycle of purification and growth begins.

Reiki is, in brief, deep relaxation brought about by increased contact with the divine energy from which, under Reiki's influence, we receive more than we could under normal circumstances. In a Reiki session, the amount of Reiki drawn is determined by the person receiving the treatment. Whoever receives Reiki energy, draws, within the given scope, the amount of life energy he needs to take in. This is a simple law which at once also defines the limits of Reiki therapy.

If a living being consciously or (as is mostly the case) unconsciously does not want any contact with the Universal Life Energy, he will not receive the flow of Reiki energy; in that case, nothing will be felt as energy drawing through the hands. The dissociation may arise from feelings of guilt or the conviction of being too "evil" or too "sinful". This "sin" or "guilt complex" is the greatest impediment to healing. If you believe you deserve your illness, you won't let anything come near you that could bring about your healing.

There is a divine spark within each human being. This spark of divine or love energy resonates perfectly with Reiki, which is of the same source and helps the individual to experience unconditional love. God loves every human being as he or she is, the murderer no less than the saint.

A life-threatening disease is a race against time. The challenge is to delay death until the sick person becomes aware of his own divine spark. Conventional medicine can fulfill this important task. Thanks to its amazing possibilities it can give this important period of time to a sick person in the case of an emergency. It can prolong life and thus give the sick person a chance to let go of his guilt complex. During this period, psychotherapeutic counseling and other physical therapies, the presence of kind, loving friends who understand the situation of the sick person, as well as naturopathy and work with the techniques of Second Degree Reiki (mental treatment) can help remove the guilt complexes which have cut the sick person off from any possibilities of healing so far.

In my experience nobody is condemned to any kind of illness unless he actually wants to be ill. What expresses itself in an illness is always a healthy but repressed need of a person manifesting in the area most accessible to him at that time. If this repressed need discovers a new area which is more easily accessible, it will manifest there. If someone has a need, for example, to experience the love of his fellow beings, and if he will not allow himself to accept this experience in a healthy way, he will sometimes choose a suitable illness as justification to then create this experience. In this way, we can also easily determine the causal factor of a person's illness. Observation of the changes in his behavior and that of his social environment during the illness provide many clues.

If the sick person is prepared, even to a modest degree, to explore new areas and spheres of experience, this very willingness will be the most important starting-point for a meaningful, promising course of treatment, as it represents his will to live, which necessarily includes the will to be healthy.

But how about the sick person's right to be ill? I am convinced we have to accept it. That is why I would no try to help anyone who categorically refuses help. Each person has his own reasons for refusing help. I will accept his refusal out of respect for his dignity as a living being, even if I am not able to understand it. A human being should have the right to determine his own fate without having to justify his choice before others.

Even if he refuses the type of help I offer, there may be someone else whose help he would gratefully accept. I will then gladly assist him to establish contact with this other healer and personally step aside. In my opinion forcing healing measures on an individual is an imposition of one's will that borders on abuse.

The Limitations of Reiki Self-Treatment

Many people study meditation techniques, oracle methods or learn Reiki because they fear confronting their own problems in interaction with others, for example during group therapy."Inner" work for such a person is simply an inward "escape". However valuable various methods may be, the attitude with which one works is all important. Methods for self-realization cannot replace direct life experience. Even Reiki cannot do that. If you are facing serious problems with yourself or others, or if your seemingly minor problems are actually of a serious nature, you should consult an experienced therapist whom you can trust. He can help you to deal with your anxieties when they arise, to support you when you believe you have failed, and show you new, life-giving ways to help you to get back on your feet. You will make faster progress in your therapy and accelerate your progress toward self-reliance if you pamper yourself with regular whole body treatment with Reiki. In this way, after having created a sound foundation by getting in touch with the true Self, continued Reiki practise will further enhance your self-growth. Everyday life will provide enough lessons for further growth once you are stabilized in a positive environment.

The same is also true of physical disorders. If you are seriously ill, it is best to consult a good allopathist, homeopath or physician specialized in naturopathy. If you attempt to cure yourself without knowing all the possible variables without proper research you could cause greater harm than good. After all, even persons with professional training in medicine or psychology will consult a colleague if they find they are seriously ill. Reiki will then act as a great support to correct treatment, and help to accelerate the healing process.

Summary
Possibilities and Limitations of Reiki Application

First Degree
Possibilities:
- Deep relaxation
- Release of blockages
- Detoxification
- Supply of universal life-force energy
- Increase of the vibrational frequency

Limitations:
- Recipient's absence or lack of receptiveness
- Channel could be limited to begin with, although channel gets stronger with time, with practise
- Regular sessions are desirable
- Cannot give distance treatment
- will need other treatments in addition to Reiki in case of serious illness.

Second Degree
Possibilities:
- all possibilities of the first degree, but with a significantly higher capacity of Reiki energy
- no immediate, close contact is necessary for the Reiki session (distance treatment)
- although unconscious blocks may exist, it is possible to release these blockages in the case of conscious willingness to receive treatment(mental treatment).

Limitations:
- deliberate refusal of healing
- channel may not be as strong at the beginning, although capacity increases with time
- might not be effective, if regular session not possible
- should not be applied as sole treatment in acute emergencies, but is an excellent support in emergency intervention
- Will need other forms of treatment in addition to Reiki in cases of serious illness

Chapter Three

Preparatory Procedures or Rituals in Reiki Whole Body Treatment

At introductory seminars for First Dgree Reiki, some Reiki teachers use formal proceduresor "rituals" before and after whole body treatment. Unfortunately there is often not enough time to explain these clearly, which is why many students forget them. As with all formal procedures, including the "Reiki rituals" it is helpful to know their meaning and use. The following may help to elucidate some of my own personal procedures.

Removing Jewelry

Nearly everyone likes to wear jewelry; precious stones, semi-precious stones, precious metals, objects made of wood or leather. However beautiful these things are, I feel that they may cause some problems on an energetic level. Metals and stones attract certain subtle energies. In (alternative) medicine, these qualities are used in therapy in order to draw "negative energies" from the body. But the capacity of these aids is limited. Precious stone therapists know by experience that they have to regularly purify stones used for healing purposes.

If they do not do so, these beautiful stones will no longer be able to heal, or at worst even "fall ill" themselves. Moreover, stones saturated with negative energies have an equivalent emanation. This is also similar with metals, glass and plastic. On the other hand, organic materials such as wood and leather are not so easily charged with negative energy from the environment.

Pieces of jewelry which we wear all day long inevitably have contact with all kinds of energy vibrations. If they have become "saturated" with energies in their environment they act like miniature jamming stations and will irritate their carriers, either more or less according to their susceptibility to subtle vibrations. Thus, your headache may disappear rather quickly if you clean your glasses regu-

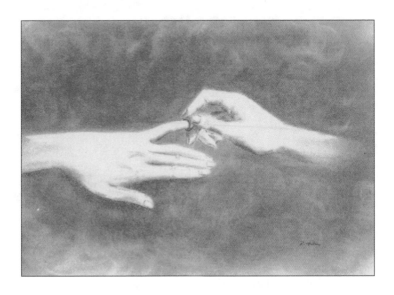

Fig. 3: Removing jewelry

larly in running water. Earrings of any shape are a special case. There are dozens of acupuncture points on the outer ear which can affect the whole body. Earrings are fixed directly beside these points and therefore transmit their interfering emission directly into the energetic channels of the body. In order to create the most disturbance-free atmosphere you should remove all jewelry. (Refer to the Appendix for information on cleaning jewelry).

Rings, chains and watches often form closed metal circuits.

As can be easily demonstrated with the pendulum or the "diamond arm test" the flow of energy in the body is reduced by such closed circuits. Being a higher form of energy than the meridian energy, the flow of Reiki energy will not be impeded. However, the subtle energy system of the body may not fully respond to Reiki energy due to impairment caused by these metal circuits.

Quartz watches even emit their own rhythm of subtle electromagnetic vibrations which can be measured electronically and through dowsing. As the human body has a different vibration frequency, yet is not unaffected by the rhythm of the quartz watch, the latter acts as a constant source of interference which the body must counteract. At least during Reiki sessions this potential interference should be excluded. If you would like to do yourself a favor apart from Reiki treatment, you might consider buying one of the attractive and reliable mechanical watches available on the market.

Naturally this advice also applies to the Reiki channel who transfers Reiki energy to his clients. The person transferring Reiki may also benefit from the energy flowing at each session. The energy flow may also be greater for the practitioner if potential sources of interference are eliminated.

Washing Your Hands

According to the New Testament, Pontius Pilot's comment on the condemnation of Christ was "I wash my hands of this whole affair, I am innocent." This is certainly not the most positive example of the symbolism of washing hands, but it contains the key word—innocence.

Apart from the obvious hygienic purpose, washing your hands also has an aesthetic meaning. Hands constantly touch a lot of things and also perspire. In the initial positions of whole body treatment they are placed directly on the face or next to it where the client will readily smell any odors and feel the hands through the highly-sensitive facial nerves. If the hands have a neutral smell and do not stick to the skin this will be more pleasant for the recipient of Reiki treatment.

Another reason for washing our hands before and after Reiki treatment is to be found on the subtle plane. The human body is surrounded by a field of energy; it has an aura. We can even see it with the Kirilian-photography method. The aura has a similar function on the subtle plane as does the skin on the grosser plane. It protects the inner energy body and provides the transfer of subtle information and energies which flow into the body and out of it. As with the surface of the skin, the aura too absorbs the imprints of those things with which it comes in contact. These imprints may cause irritation in sensitive individuals, but running water washes them away. Washing your hands after a Reiki session helps you to rid yourself of the imprints which you may have taken on from the treated person.

If for some reason water is not available, you can also pass your hands on both sides of a candle flame. This will also effect an energetic cleansing.

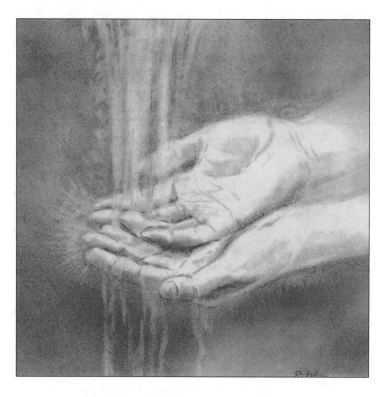

Fig. 4: Washing hands

The Invocation

Before starting with whole body treatment I join my hands as in prayer on the heart level, and ask mentally or aloud that I may act as a Reiki channel and I ask for the healing of the person on whom I am going to place my hands. Then I raise my hands to my forehead, bow my head and my upper body and lower my hands again to the heart level.

This ritual is a gesture of respect for the person to whom I will now channel Reiki. Through it I am at the same time accepting myself and him or her in the core of my being.

The joining of hands represents the union of my yin and yang parts, the bright and dark sides on the level of my heart. On this level the process of loving acceptance of the world, of human beings and of my Self takes place. Without the invocation at this level of awareness, real acceptance of reality is not possible. Here the demands and actualities of the material world unite with those of the subtle spheres. Through this part of the ritual I am symbolically accepting myself in a very loving manner. Through this procedure I am able to make deeper contact with another person as well, and accept him lovingly with all his faults and both his light and dark sides. This process of acceptance is a level of pure feeling which cannot be evoked mentally, but is cultivated through reverence or respect for what some may call "Christ energy" or "true Self".

After this symbolic union with love, I raise my hands to my forehead, to my Third Eye, which gives me the knowledge and acceptance of my personal path. This level is only accessible to those who have fully accepted themselves. Through this acceptance I also understand that my path will not always proceed according to plan; I let go of my attachment to my desire to control, and turn inward to my true Self which really guides me as it does all humanity.

I joyfully accept that my development may actually take quite a different turn than what I had expected. Nevertheless I trust that it will be perfect in accordance to the lessons I need to learn. This positive, open-minded attitude represents the epitome of true faith.

Whenever I accept myself fully, I can also then accept another person fully. I thus accept his freedom of choice to use the Reiki energy as he chooses and not as I think he should. Simultaneously with the gesture of the hands, I bow my head and thus surrender the

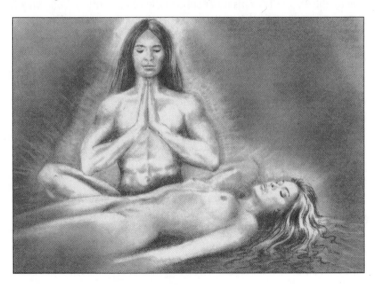

Fig. 5: The invocation

35

responsibility for this growth to the Universal Spirit, Christ, Buddha—or however you choose to describe supreme perfection. I fully acknowledge the dignity of the human being before me. Although some of his problems may be more evident than mine at the moment, I am aware that this person is no less valuable, wise or important for the world than I am myself. His problems or illness make him no less perfect, they are only a reflection of the lessons he needs to learn.

Smoothing out the Aura

Before laying your hands on the body you may smooth out the aura of your client. To do this, you should sit by his side, place your left hand on your hara and with your right hand, palm facing downwards, stroke along the mid-line of the body from head to toe at a distance of about 8 inches. Having arrived at the feet, place your hand in a vertical position and pass it closely over your body back toward the head. There you start again. I repeat this procedure three times. After completing the Reiki session you may place your left hand on the hara (abdomen) or the sacrum (lower back) of your client and repeat the same procedure.

I use this technique to establish contact. Your client will perceive you on the threshold of his inner subtle field of perception. You "knock at his door", as it were, and ask to be allowed to enter. You don't want to kick it down and say, "look out, here I come!". By placing your left (receiving) hand on your hara and establishing contact with the right (giving hand) you can convey your centeredness. With deeper Reiki contact you may perceive the union of Self; yourself and the other, totally unmasked. While these processes mostly take place more or less unconsciously, they are nonetheless real and important! By moving your flat hand in the direction of the flow of his aura (from head to feet), you convey your presence everywhere, smoothing out superficial energy build-ups and stimulating a harmonious flow of energy in the aura.

After the Reiki session you may repeat the same procedure as a closure. This time you can place your left hand on the client's hara or sacrum, (his center point in martial arts). In this way you help the person feel his or her own source of energy and illustrate that he is not dependent on your energy.

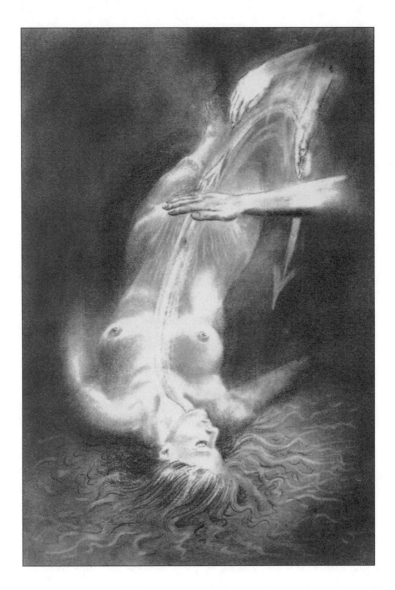

Fig. 6:
Smoothing out the aura

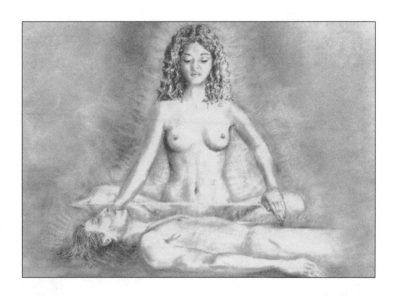

Fig. 7: Positive energy stroke

The Energy Stroke

At the end of the session you may carry out a fast stroke from the pelvis to the crown above the middle of the body with your hand placed vertically.

This technique supplies the whole body with energy from the root chakra. It was used by the famous healer Franz Anton Mesmer at the beginning of the last century to help bring people out of a fainting spell or also to supply them with energy. You can experiment with the amazing effect of this simple method by means of the arm test used in kinesiology.

For this test instruct a partner to stretch his arm out horizontally. You then press the arm down with a fast movement. Make a mental note of his power of resistance. Now you make a negative energy stroke on your partner with your hand along the mid-line of his body from head to pelvis. Then check the strength of his arm again. In most cases it will be significantly diminished. If you then do a positive stroke (that is, from the pelvis to the crown), your partner will in most cases respond with greater strength. If you would like to learn more about this test refer to John Diamond's "Your Body Does not Lie" (see Bibliography). Perhaps you will wonder how important these procedures are with regard to Reiki treatment.

Basically this depends on your own approach and on that of your client. You may be familiar, for example, with the effects of prayer on healing. As in prayer, it is always your conscious participation which determines the final result of any effort. If your own ritual or procedure is meaningful to you, perform it with the utmost awareness; however don't force yourself to do anything which feels inappropriate to you. This would be to your disadvantage.

If you are not attached to your own rituals (which is preferable) it is better to use your intuition to tune to the needs of your client and see if indeed your "rituals" or procedure are appropriate to his belief system. If he knows your rituals or procedures and their significance, let him make the decision if you are not sure. The basic procedures for Reiki are easily intelligible. For example everyone will be able to easily understand the significance of washing your hands.

It is best not to blindly perform "rituals" or procedures which have no meaning for you. If they appear totally meaningless to you, don't do them! Perhaps a time may come in the future when certain rituals may seem appropriate. When done with conscious awareness, you may use any of the described procedures for your personal growth. Even such a simple thing as washing your hands can be significant. What does cleanliness mean, after all? Is it superfluous for you to create calm and cleanliness around you if you want to experience your center, or is it just a simple act of hygiene?

Rituals basically work like a lever. Put a little of your energy into them, and you put cosmic laws into operation which then ensure that a lot of energy starts moving. Reiki itself needs no rituals. It is always flowing! What these rituals really do is help you become more aware, and thus consciously open up to the process which Reiki initiates. In some cases, they may also speed up the effect of Reiki, having made you or your client more receptive. Therefore, Reiki rituals are an important element of Reiki-Do.

Procedures after the
Reiki Session

After finishing whole body treatment, you may smooth out the aura again and use the energy stroke. I normally give thanks for the ability to transfer the Reiki energy, wash my hands and sometimes advise my client to drink a lot of water, take a shower, avoid alcohol, get more rest, or whatever seems appropriate at the time.

Summary

Suggestions for rituals in Reiki whole body treatment

Remove *jewelry and quartz watches* to eliminate potential interference in the flow of Reiki energy or its harmonizing effect.

Washing your hands to effect a physical as well as subtle cleansing so that your client is not disturbed.

The main *invocation*, according to the hermetic law is "as above so below". By setting the ego to one side and making contact with the true Self, you open yourself to a greater receptivity of Reiki.

Smoothing out the aura is suitable for establishing gentle contact with the client, stimulating various functions and is also appropriate for terminating the contact at the end of the treatment.

The *energy stroke* has a strengthening and stimulating effect.

Chapter Four

The Advantages of Reiki Whole Body Treatment

Neither a person's inner being nor his physical body can be dissected into component parts functioning independently of each other. Every organ, every cell, every manifestation of life is directly or indirectly interconnected with all others, is supported by them and in turn supports them. If disorder occurs in a specific part of the body, its causes and effects exist in other parts as well. If you suffer from indigestion, for instance, it will affect the rest of your body in the course of time due to the incomplete assimilation of food. Gradually, wastes will accumulate in the fatty tissue, the muscles, the blood vessels and the joints. Your eliminating organs will constantly have to work overtime in order to stop the flood of toxins. If they begin to fail over a longer period of time, some form of inflammation is likely to develop. This will impose a strain on your lymphatic system which is responsible for eliminating toxins arising in the course of inflammation. As a result of this pathological development you start feeling sluggish and prefer to stay at home instead of engaging in the sports you used to enjoy. Your lymphatic system, however, needs exercise to function properly, so inactivity will additionally impair its function. You may then soon have trouble with your tonsils or irritation of the appendix (the appendix is also part of the lymphatic system). The immune system is then affected and becomes unable to cope with the situation and easily breaks down when attacked by the next 'flu bug. If you then proceed to launch a "chemical counterattack" with antibiotics, pain killers and cortisone, some even more serious health setbacks are sure to occur.

Even Reiki treatment of the inflamed lymph nodes (tonsils) in the throat will not be very helpful and will only result, if at all, in some superficial recovery. The simple reason is that the cause for the excessive burden has not been removed.

Even if one cause has been determined, and this can be especially difficult with long-term chronic conditions, there will be other contributing causes due to the links between bodily functions. In most cases, several suppressed inflammations are probably smoldering in several areas of the body.

Especially in this kind of situation you should not be concerned with the various causes, but rather give extensive whole body treatment over a long period of time. By way of the different positions through which Reiki is conveyed during treatment of about 90 minutes all the important organs will be supplied with the revitalizing energy of Reiki in a coordinated sequence. In this way, the responsiveness of the body is slowly and gradually restored and the energy channels and metabolic systems will regain their conductivity and ability to cope with toxic burdens and stress.

This process is very important. Nearly all naturopathic treatments attempt to stimulate the healing reactions of the body. In many cases the body is burdened by toxins and cannot properly respond to the self-healing stimulus. In homeopathic medicine special remedies are employed to enable the organism to respond to the stimulus. Reiki whole body treatment solves this problem in a much easier way. Without any experimenting, the metabolism is stimulated, which in turn activates thorough cleansing. With time the body regains its responsiveness all on its own.

Whole body treatment has another advantage, as it directly and extensively regenerates the subtle energy channels and metabolic systems. Naturopathic treatments often fail simply because of the body's lack of capacity to channel the activated energies. Actually, they often present a strain at first, a strain under which the body may collapse entirely.

The liver, kidneys, and heart may not be able to take the additional strain caused by the therapy and may fail to function. Reiki rebuilds this ability to cope with strain and in many cases even very quickly. It allows the body to harmoniously utilize the healing responses that have been activated.

If the body is weakened by the process of healing, Reiki whole body treatment will help to supply the energies needed to cope with the illness. Therefore, Reiki is a beneficial support for all natural healing methods. During any holistic therapy it should be applied as an additional aid, as it will contribute to the recovery and strengthening of the entire organism.

In forms of treatment involving chemical drugs (allopathic remedies), Reiki can reduce side effects and help the body to recover from this "chemical assault" once the course of medication is completed. Reiki whole body treatment is particularly helpful after chemotherapy for cancer. The same is also true for follow-up treatments after an operation. After an operation the body is weakened greatly. It has to form new tissue, cope with the shock of an operation and may also be forced to combat germs. Often there is severe pain. Scars which have not been properly dealt with may later result in new complaints. Reiki whole body treatment during this period supplies the body with additional life energy and thus helps it to cope with the added strain. If Reiki is regularly applied immediately after an operation there will be little or no pain. The healing process in the tissue is speeded up and scars treated with Reiki are often hardly visible later and will not cause problems in the future. What is important here is the regularity of the Reiki sessions. This alone will ensure lasting success.

Reiki Whole Body Treatment for Personal Growth

So chronic disease is not a relevant issue for you? All the better! Especially people who already enjoy good health will gain tremendous benefit from Reiki whole body treatment.

When it is regularly applied it enhances a healthy ability to respond appropriately to your environment on all levels. By developing greater openness you will be able to allow more things to touch you. You will face people and the world without stress. In this way, you will gain more and more self-confidence. With time you will begin to live your life more intensely and gain more from your experiences. Regular Reiki whole body treatment also has a prophylactic effect and enables the body to eliminate germs before they affect your health. Latent capabilities will be activated and you will be able to learn more easily and apply whatever you have learned more effectively.

Hard to believe? Just try it yourself! These positive changes which are often found after any thorough cleansing or stimulation of the physical body can also be observed with other natural healing processes. Once an individual no longer has to waste precious energy unproductively, coping with blockages and chronic complaints, a tremendous potential for personal growth will automatically open up.

Reiki Whole Body Treatment and Rejuvenation

Naturally, you may also use Reiki for rejuvenation on all levels. Reiki energy lays no claim to being a "fountain of youth", but it is much more effective and inexpensive than many of the miracle drugs, panaceas and potions available on the market. Reiki whole body treatment will not cause any damage, a danger that does exist with preparations that are not necessarily closely attuned to the particular need of the individual.

Reiki energy gradually improves the circulation which means a more balanced functioning of the skin, so that some of your tiny wrinkles may disappear. Moreover, thorough activation of the metabolism including the functions of detoxification also improves the tone of the connective tissue and muscles. Naturally these processes do require a certain amount of time. If you believe you are worth it and are willing to take this time, I am certain you will be very pleased with the results of Reiki treatment.

In the majority of cases Reiki whole body treatment will not cause any unduly severe healing reactions. If blockages are removed in any area of the body and energies are released, subsequent Reiki treatment will ensure harmonious distribution of these energies so that they do not cause intense reactions. Nevertheless, dramatic healing reactions may arise in the course of Reiki treatment. Therefore specific Reiki treatment should only be given by experienced and qualified practitioners.

Summary
The advantages of Reiki whole body treatment

– Recovery of responsiveness
– Thorough cleansing
– Additional life energy
– Safe, holistic treatment
– No unilateral release of blocked energy

Chapter Five

The Positions
of Reiki Whole Body Treatment
and its Effects on the Organic
and Subtle Bodies

In this chapter I will present a practical sequence of positions for whole body treatment. I have essentially adopted this sequence from my Reiki master Brigitte Müller and have added some positions I acquired from other Reiki practitioners along with some I adopted in my own practise. While this sequence has proved very successful, there are many other options. Other Reiki masters often proceed differently in whole body treatment, which is no less effective and in certain cases even more appropriate. It is not my intention to present one and only correct form of whole body treatment (I believe there no such thing, since every human being is different), but rather offer you a well-coordinated sequence along with some guidance from which you can develop your own repertoire.

In my experience it is important to initially understand why a specific sequence of positions is beneficial. Eventually, as you gain experience and develop your own inner knowledge, the details will become less important. Once your intuition is awakened you will not need to rely so strongly on rational concepts as you did to begin with. If you work a lot with Reiki, this development will come by itself. It may take some time until this stage is reached, and for most people the preliminary and later concurrent intellectual preoccupation with fixed forms and their inherent logic is simply necessary. You will know by your positive results whether you still require the structures presented in this book and when you will be able to depend solely on your intuition. From this point of view, my system becomes superfluous the more you work with it - and that is the way it should be.

But let's start at the beginning. The following is a description of the complete sequence I use in most Reiki sessions. You may use it as a whole or in parts according to your needs.

Before Reiki Whole Body Treatment

First of all, you might ask inwardly for permission to treat the person seeking help. Consider the responsibility connected with it and determine whether you are qualified to take it. Whenever there is even the slightest reason to assume that your client suffers from serious physical or mental illness, and you are neither a physician nor a non-medical practitioner, for instance, you should immediately assign the responsibility to other more qualified persons. If you want to apply Reiki along with some medical treatment or psychotherapy, you might enquire as to whether and how your client is being treated with drugs and have them ask their physician or psychotherapist if any doubts remain. If that is not possible, you might initially limit your Reiki work to fewer treatments. You will find more advice on this in Chapters Two and Six.

If you feel clear about his or her situation you can proceed. It is important to obtain a time commitment from your client. Are you also willing to commit time? Are you willing to deal with some of your own issues which may come up as a reaction to the other's process? Your development may be speeded up as well. Are you ready to take this exciting step in your own development as well? If you make yourself available as a Reiki channel frequently, you can expect a definite acceleration in your own development. Are you willing to take this leap now?

After all these considerations, you can then focus on how you would like to proceed with treatment. The proper sequence for hand positions according to the client needs are presented in this chapter and Chapter Seven and may subsequently be determined in consultation with a physician or therapist. According to the scope of your own qualifications you may make your own diagnosis and perform Reiki treatment on this basis.

Questions of whole body treatment

After you have clarified your own position, the forthcoming Reiki sessions will raise further questions which also need to be clarified. First of all you should clarify whether you might want to limit whole body treatment. In the case of very weak persons and small children treatment might be shortened, for instance, to a period of about 20 minutes. You might also apply shorter treatments with fewer positions to persons taking drugs (allopathic medication) (see Chapter Twelve). If your client has a disposition for energy build-ups, manifesting as headaches, for instance, as extraordinarily severe complaints during or before the menses in women, certain positions may be omitted and the regions of the body affected by those complaints only given indirect treatment. In other cases you may need to focus on specific areas in conducting whole body treatment and specifically channel Reiki energy to especially needy areas. Possibly some partial treatment (for instance, chakra balancing or short treatment) may be advisable, which may actually have the effect of whole body treatment. Perhaps you may have to consider specific Reiki work such as emergency measures (first aid), elimination of clearly defined blockages such as scars, or local, limited inflammation, or chronic tension in certain part of the body. In many instances you will need to support Reiki work by supplementary measures such as the use of precious stones, fragrances, sounds, counseling, body-work, diet or other therapeutic measures. As in the previous questions, here too you must ask yourself whether you are qualified to make the respective decision and assume the responsibility for carrying out the appropriate measures.

More than a mere secondary consideration

You might consider a friendly chat with your client before or after treatment. Or would you prefer to say something during sessions if necessary? This depends each individual case. On some days silence may be best. You will sense if it is appropriate to speak, but at all times keep in mind the importance of a quiet, peaceful atmosphere.

"Rituals" after the Reiki session

After completing whole body treatment, you might again smooth out the aura and use the energy stroke. I always give thanks for having been allowed to transfer Reiki energy, wash my hands and perhaps advise the client to drink more water, shower, avoid alcohol, get more rest or take other appropriate measures.

The Reiki Positions

Each of the hand positions in whole body treatment have a specific significance. It is not important to imitate them exactly. It will serve the purpose if your hands are simply placed on the indicated parts of the body. Moreover, it does not matter whether a position is covered by your right or left hand, because Reiki is non-polar energy. Clothing, plaster casts or blankets do not impede Reiki energy. However, some people like to have direct body contact and in such cases it is advisable to eliminate superfluous "obstacles". If there are open wounds, burns, boils or similar symptoms, you should not lay your hands directly on the body, but place them about four inches above the corresponding reflex zones or acupuncture points. As a general rule; the more distant the reflex zones treated are from the target area, the greater and more fluid effects Reiki will have.

The following section presents various Reiki positions and specifies the organs in the areas of the body the individual positions act on. The most important indications are provided with additional information wherever necessary. At the end of the book you will find an alphabetical index of symptoms telling you which positions general experience has shown to be most appropriate for their treatment.

Positions on the Head

Position 1:

Place your hands in a parallel position to the right and left of the nose, from the forehead to the region of the top teeth.

The eyes, frontal and nasal sinuses, teeth, pituitary gland (control of the inner secretory glands should always be included in treatment in all glandular disorders; best of all, before Reiki work on the respective gland); pineal gland, sixth chakra (Third Eye), reflex zones for all important organs (the entire body is reflected in the face).

Fatigue/stress; cold complaints of the nasal and frontal sinuses; eye diseases; weakness/addiction problems; allergies; discontent. Basic position for chronic diseases of every type.

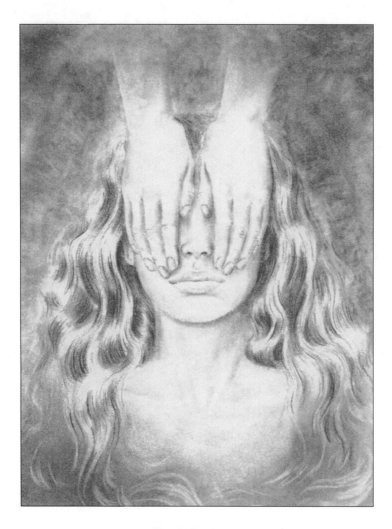

Fig. 8: Position 1

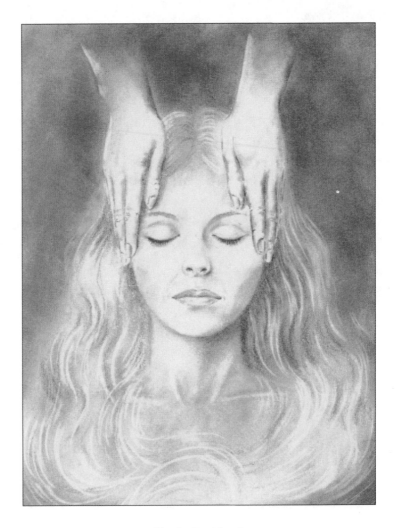

Fig. 9: Position 2

Position 2:

The hands are placed on the temples with the finger tips reaching to
the cheekbones.

Eye muscles and eye nerves; halves of the brain

Balancing the two halves of the brain (emotion and reason); useful in case of stress/difficulty in learning/lack of concentration and
whenever a person is too strongly governed by his emotions or by
reason. Colds, headache.

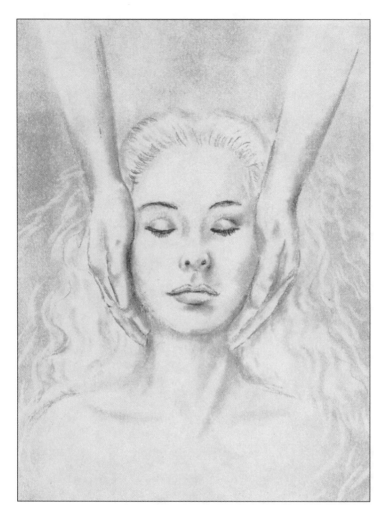

Fig. 10: Position 3

Position 3:

The hands are placed on the ears.

Ears; organs of equilibrium; pharyngeal region

As there are dozens of acupuncture points on the outer and inner ear, this is a basic position for diseases of every type. Disorders of the sense of balance. Diseases of the nasal and pharyngeal region, colds, acute loss of hearing, states of confusion.

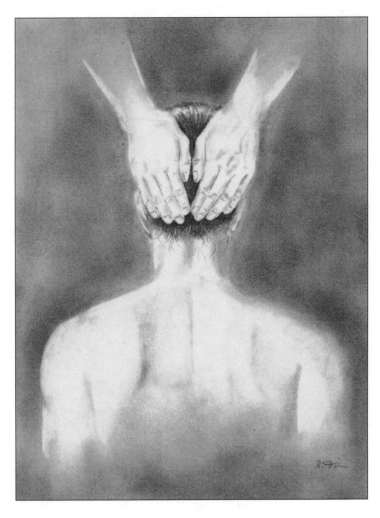

Fig. 11: Position 4

Position 4:

The hands cup the back of the head, the fingertips are placed on the medulla oblongata (the soft spot you can feel if you pass your fingers along the mid-line of the head to the neck; about halfway the hard bone ends and changes into a soft depression. This is the location of the medulla).

Reflex zones for the main chakras one to four; brain; medulla oblongata (extended spinal cord); large intestine, triple heater, gall bladder, and control meridian (governor vessel).

Relaxation. Headache, eye diseases, colds, abdominal complaints, anxiety, blockages in the sixth chakra; asthma; hyperventilation; circulatory complaints; sneezing; nausea; chronic "swallowing the wrong way".

Position 5:

The hands cover the front section of the neck. Do not touch the neck as this could cause fear in some people.

Thyroid, parathyroid gland, larynx, vocal cords, lymph nodes, fifth chakra.

Metabolic diseases, weight problems, anorexia, stuttering, anxiety; palpitation; poor posture, chronic tension of the legs, pelvic area, and shoulder muscles.Blood pressure; repressed aggression or aggressions that have been too intensely acted out. Behavioral and communicative disorders. Sore throat; tonsillitis; hoarseness; insecurity.

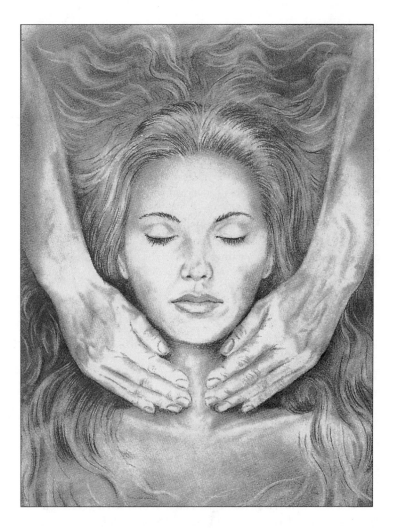

Fig. 12: Position 5

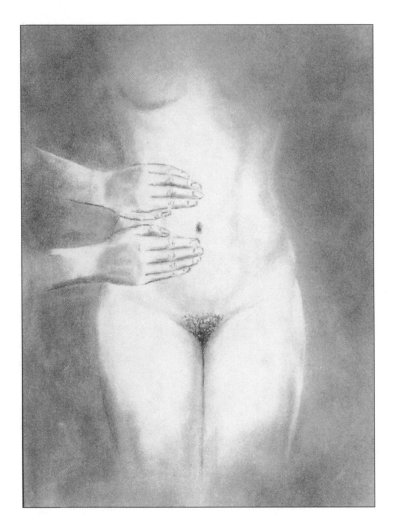

Fig. 13: Position 6

Positions on the Trunk
Position 6:

One hand is placed on the lowest ribs on the right side, the other hand directly below.

Liver and gall bladder

Diseases of liver and gall bladder; digestive trouble; haemorrhoids; excessive and repressed aggressions; high blood pressure; metabolic disease; detoxification.

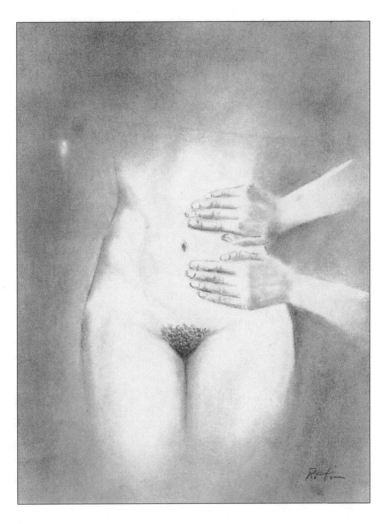

Fig. 14: Position 7

Position 7:

Exact mirror-image of osition six. Place your hands on the left lower ribs and directly below.

Parts of the pancreas; spleen; bowels.

Diabetes (also see special elbow position); diseases of pancreas and spleen; disposition for infections (tendency to inflammation); formation of blood (red corpuscles); indigestion.

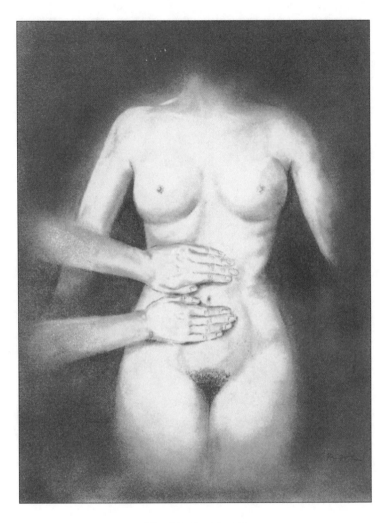

Fig. 15: Position 8

Position 8:

One hand is placed above the navel, the other below it.

Solar plexus, stomach, third chakra, digestive organs, hara.

Anxiety; inner harmony; gastro-intestinal disease; nausea; heartburn; bloated feeling; promotes digestion; haemorrhoids; increases vitality; pride and feeling of inferiority; metabolic diseases; depression.

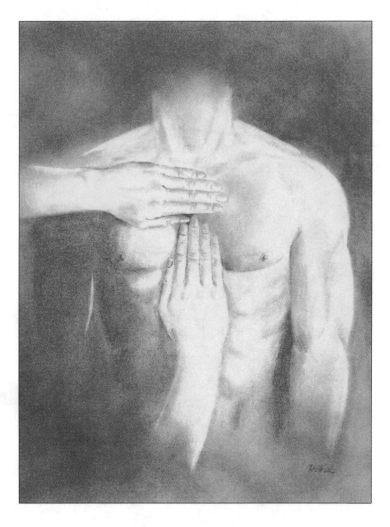

Fig. 16: Position 9

Position 9:

One hand is placed across the thymus, the other hand at a right angle below and between the breasts (with both hands together forming a "T")

Thymus; heart; lungs; fourth chakra.

Strengthening of the immune system; heart trouble; lymphatic system; deafness; excessive emotion or lack of emotion; lung disease; general weakness; depression.

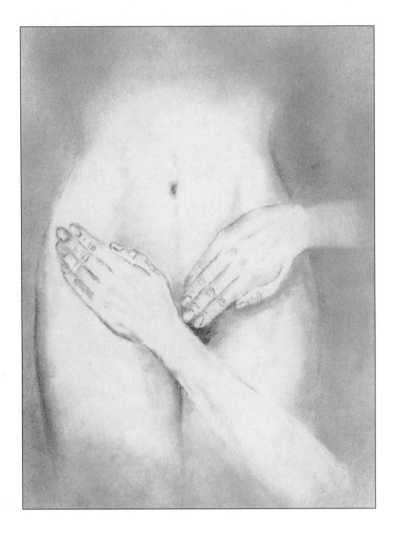

Fig. 17: Position 10

Position 10:

The balls of the thumb are each placed on the ridges of the pelvic bones, the tips of the hands close to each other at the pubic bone, forming a "V".

Urogenital organs; intestines; appendix; first and second chakras.

Diseases of the urogenital system; breast tumors; climacteric complaints; digestive trouble; fear of physical closeness, allergies (main position); general weakness; convalescence; sexual problems; weight problems; anorexia; circulation; strengthening the immune system; lack of will to live and of joy of life.

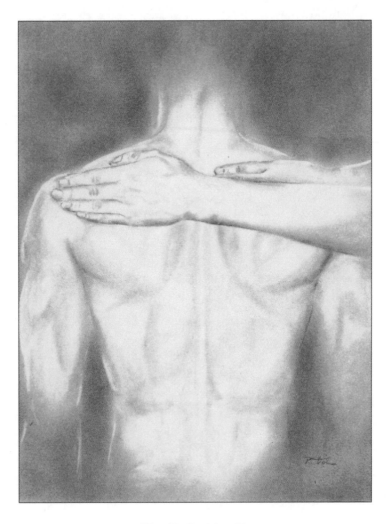

Fig. 18: Position 11

Positions on the Back
Position 11:

The hands are placed between the shoulders and the shoulder blades.

Minor chakras (responsibility); neck and shoulder muscles; triple heater, small intestine, large intestine, bladder and gall bladder meridian.

Headache; tension in the shoulders and neck; problems with responsibility (feels responsible for everything and everyone/always worried/never wants to shoulder responsibility)

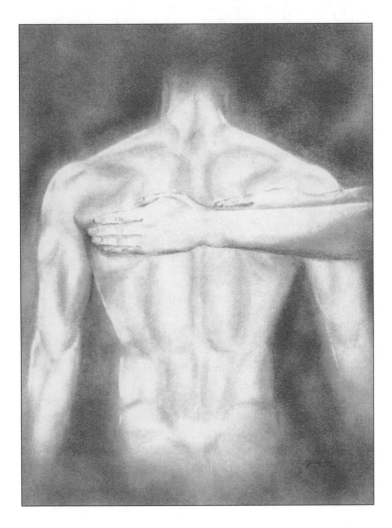

Fig. 19: Position 12

Position 12:

Hands are placed on the shoulder blades.

Lung; heart; small intestine and bladder meridian

Lung and heart diseases; difficulty to admit feelings/totally at the mercy of one's feelings; manic depression.

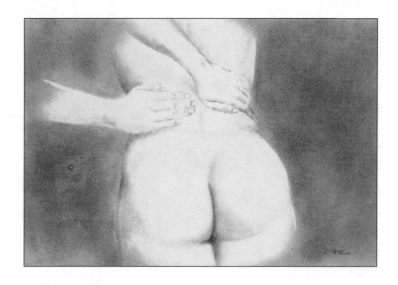

Fig. 20: Position 13

Position 13:

The hands are placed on the lower ribs above the kidney.

Adrenal glands, kidneys.

Stress; every type of problem in partnerships and relationships; kidney diseases; allergies; shock (this position is very important to prevent kidney failure after a shock!); detoxification; cleansing therapies; sexual problems; fear of physical closeness; fear of heights and falling; difficulty in sharing feelings.

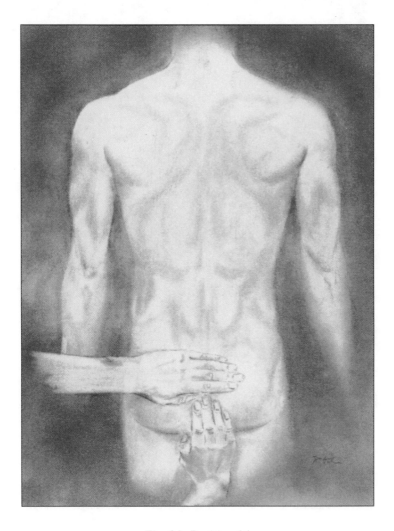

Fig. 21: Position 14

Position 14:

One hand is placed across the sacral plate (bone plate above the fold of the buttocks), the other hand vertically below (with a little more pressure).

First chakra; intestines; urogenital system; sciatica.

Strengthening; haemorrhoids (only symptomatic effect!); digestive trouble; fissures and enteritis; sciatic complaints; diseases of the urogenital system.

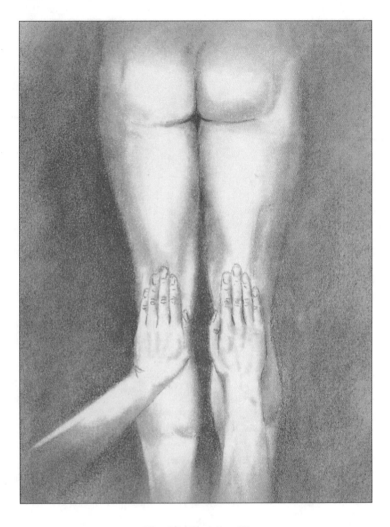

Fig. 22: Position 15

Position 15:

The hands cover the hollows of the knee.

Minor chakras (flexible adjustment to all situations of life; capacity for learning; criticism); knee joint; meniscus; kneecap; bursa.

Joint damage; sports injuries; blockages affecting the flow of energy from the feet to the root chakra.

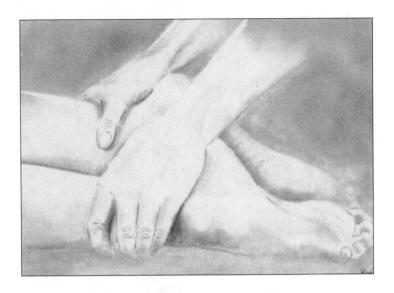

Fig. 23: Position 16

Position 16:

The hands are placed around the ankles.

    Joints; reflex zones for the pelvic organs.

    Joint damage; blockages impairing the flow of energy to the root chakra; diseases in the entire pelvic region.

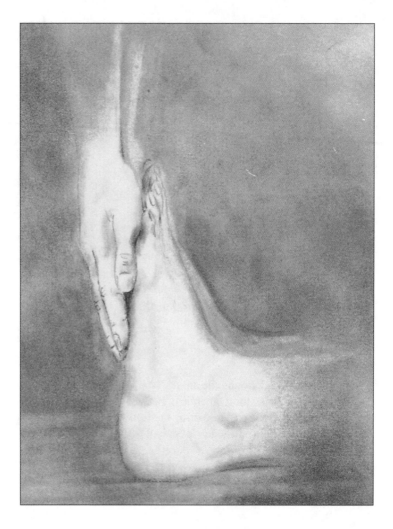

Fig. 24: Position 17

Position 17

The hands are placed on the soles of the feet, the big toes must be covered from the tips.
Reflex zones for all organs; stomach, liver, kidney and gall bladder meridian.

Grounding of all chakras and body regions; headache; strengthening of the root chakra and the aura. Especially important for oversensitive people. To be recommended after coma, anaesthesia, every type of shock. Effective whole body treatment can be given through the soles of the feet, the tops of the feet and the ankles.

Special Positions

Diabetes: The hands are placed on the elbows; give regular treatment for at least 10 minutes respectively.

Hip joint problems: Place hands laterally to the right and the left on the hips. Apply regular treatment over a long period of time; if possible, no treatment should last less than ten minutes.

Multiple sclerosis: Place both hands on the top of the head. Treat regularly and during episodes (not less than ten minutes per session).

Sciatica: One hand covers the sacral plate, the other is placed on the sole of one foot. Always treat both legs and carry out treatment on a regular basis if possible (at least ten minutes per session).

Heart attack (also for aftercare over a long period of time!): Only let Reiki energy flow in above or below the heart; never place the hands directly over the heart! (In case of heart attack, call a physician immediately!)

Please note: Reiki is a supplement to first aid measures. On no account can Reiki replace these measures. This reservation also applies to all diseases.

The healing effect of Reiki can be very roughly "calculated" as follows: Period of treatment x frequency of treatments x Reiki capacity of the treating Reiki channel x subconscious readiness to grow of the person treated x divine will. Without the Universal Spirit nothing will work at all!

However, the Universal Spirit rarely has any objection to healing. Most obstacles to healing are of human origin.

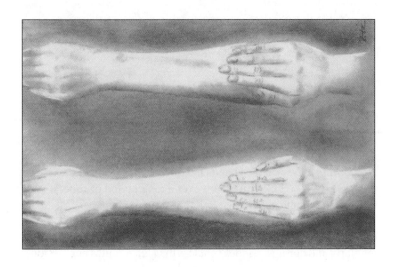

Fig. 25: Special position for "diabetes"

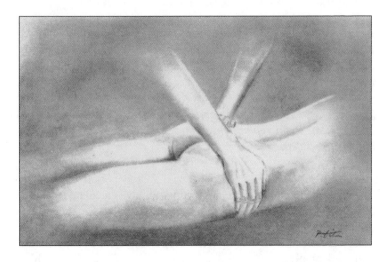

Fig. 26: Special position for "hip joints"

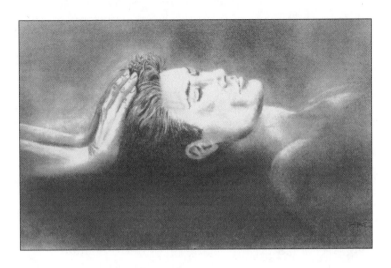

Fig. 27: Special position for "multiple sclerosis"

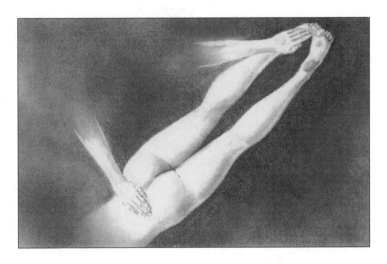

Fig. 28: Special position for "sciatica"

Chapter Six

Specific Reiki Applications

My main objective in this chapter is to give basic information on specific Reiki applications. Positions suitable for special purposes can be studied in the summary at the end of the previous chapter. But before giving specific Reiki treatment within the framework of whole body treatment, or applying it without special positions, you might consider the following question:

> *"Why do I believe that specific Reiki work within the framework of whole body treatment is appropriate in this case?"*

Specific application of Reiki energy is certainly appropriate for clearly defined blockages and acute symptoms. As a general rule; blockages presenting obstacles to receiving Reiki (i.e. you don't feel the energy drawing) can be loosened up before giving further Reiki. These blockages may be chronic and usually feel cold; nothing seems to pass through. These are generally old traumas, shocks to the system which have not been dealt with and similar blockages. Other areas which draw a lot of energy and feel very hot to the touch will be loosened up after whole body treatment. These "hot" blockages are acute or sub acute energy build-ups that are discharged without too much difficulty but which sometimes have a tendency to tie up energy again after the initial release because another, yet deeper blockage may continue to exist. If you are not sure where to concentrate, you may give whole body treatment before addressing any blockages and not concern yourself with determining the main areas of treatment right at the beginning.

As these build-ups are released, crying, laughter, rage, sadness or other feelings may surge up in your client. It is good to be open to these releases. Also take care that your client does not leave the session with a blockage which, though loosened up, is only partially and not completely acted out. He may be otherwise be overwhelmed by feelings that surge up and possibly have to face a critical situation without any assistance a short time later. Often it is difficult to determine how fast a blockage is dissolving and how much energy is being released in the process. What is important is that the energy released is integrated, which is evident when the client is able to accept his feelings. It can be a challenge if someone becomes aware of issues that have so far been suppressed, and he or she finds it difficult to deal with this confrontation. Usually Reiki on its own is not recommended for this type of integrative work, especially as it would simply require too much time. The various methods of psychological therapies such as rebirthing and various forms of body work are suitable for this day and age of emotional release work. Working with rose quartz can also be of help.

On the organic level, it might be appropriate to give specific treatment to problem areas so that weakened organs and vessels are supplied with additional life-force energy. There are special positions, for instance, for diabetes, multiple sclerosis, whiplash injury etc. Please refer to Chapter Five for more detailed information.

"Why do I believe that in this case specific Reiki work without other additional forms of treatment is appropriate?"

This question must be answered in the affirmative, especially in emergencies. Reiki can be very useful in emergencies; its application can even be of decisive importance and help bridge the gap until medical assistance arrives, e.g. for treating kidney shock, for stopping bleeding, for calming, etc.
It can, however also be helpful for minor injuries such as minor burns, cuts, insect bites, sore feet and so forth. Minor health disorders such as cramp when playing sport, stomach pains, nausea, headache and a sore throat can first be treated with Reiki without resorting to drugs.

"What other tools will I need to support my specific Reiki work?"

A "confidence building" discussion is always helpful before a Reiki session, and the use of fragrances and music helps create a positive atmosphere. Specific measures which help the client become more receptive, such as releasing energy blocks through techniques such as faith healing, work with precious stones, massage (with essential oils), work with mantras or vowels and affirmations are also useful aids (e.g. "I am ready to receive love", "I accept myself as I am". "I am whole" ... or other appropriate affirmations). It may be important to talk to the client after the Reiki session or shed light on released feelings. Selecting a stone suitable for the development that has been initiated (see Chapter Nine) or a fragrance (see Chapter Eleven) might

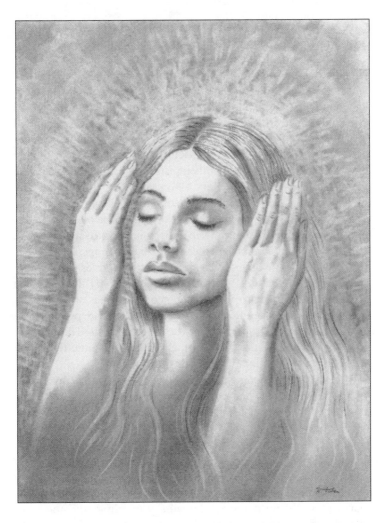

Fig. 29: Relaxation exercise with Reiki

often be very helpful. If you realize that your client needs additional assistance after your session which you cannot give yourself or are not allowed to give due to statutory regulations, you should refer him to a qualified therapist for further assistance.

How do I measure up to the responsibility involved in giving Reiki? What is my legal status in this particular case?"

If you are not able to find a definitive answer to the first question, you may simply ask an oracle or talk with your client about your uncertainty. By doing so you may gain additional confidence and also enhance the client's trust. Often some clarifying discussion will actually suffice to solve this problem. However. if you feel your client's illness is far beyond your capacity, you should consider sharing the responsibility with another therapist who might be more capable in this particular case.

If you are yourself a holistic practitioner of natural therapeutics or a physician, you will be well aware of your scope of competence. If you are in a profession (physical therapist or massage therapist, for instance) that administers therapeutic applications in the wider sense, the legal boundaries of your therapeutic activities will be more narrowly set, but at the same time also fairly clearly defined. As a private person (this also includes someone who has some professional therapeutic training, but no state license) you are prohibited to do therapeutic work, especially on a commercial basis. This prohibition covers both the medical and the psychotherapeutic field. You are liable to prosecution if you work in this sector.

Naturally no one would have any objection, of course, if you help your partner in case of minor health disorders or if you transmit Reiki to your children. And it is not a legal offence either to support friends or relatives with it. As soon as you take money for your services, however, difficulties arise. You should inform yourself thoroughly about the legal aspects by studying the respective laws pertaining to non-medical practitioners.

The specific application of Reiki energy by laymen should primarily serve the prevention and treatment of minor common complaints, which is much better for the body and more in keeping with nature than simply taking the most convenient medication. However, serious problems should be dealt with by a qualified licensed therapist. The information given here is meant to assist and inspire each of the latter in his or her own work with Reiki. Naturally, you may also inform yourself about all the possibilities of Reiki application in your own interest. This knowledge might be important to you in future emergencies.

Summary
Specific Reiki applications

Specific Reiki work is appropriate:
in emergencies; for treating minor diseases and disorders; for specific release of energy blockages; for strengthening certain organs or vessels.

It is recommended:
that you consider supporting measures, thus creating a state of receptiveness to the Reiki treatment before the session and ensuring the harmonious integration of the energies released from previous blocks after the session.

It is further recommended:
that you consider your qualifications and are conversant with the general legal conditions, clarifying whether you are able or allowed to take legal responsibility for any treatment and its repercussions before treatment is actually given.

Chapter Seven

Various Methods for Tracing Disturbances in the Subtle Energy System

It is sometimes important to determine as exactly as possible the main areas requiring treatment and the problem areas on the subtle plane (etheric body) before a Reiki session. There are quite a few very effective methods for this purpose. Some are presented below.

If you work frequently with Reiki, you will develop more and more sensitivity; your hands in particular will become increasingly sensitive with time. In this way you will acquire access to imprints on the energetic plane. The following exercise will help you to sensitize your hands more quickly. You begin by keeping them apart at a distance of about 20 inches, with the palms facing each other. You then take about five minutes to bring the hands together very slowly. Feel into your palms and observe the changes taking place during this process. If you do this simple exercise daily for a few weeks, your perceptive faculty will quickly increase.

But how will you use your perceptions? How can they be interpreted?

I am afraid there's no ready-made solution for that. There are many things you have to experience yourself first before you will be able to interpret and evaluate them properly. But there are certain similar sensations that are experienced by many people and thereby form a key for proper interpretation. From your own experience you will have to examine if this key is also useful for you. You will have to observe whether and in what way your perceptions deviate from this key. After all, it is your own perception that matters, for it represents your individual access to information on the subtle level of your clients. First we will examine the most common perceptions and discuss their possible significance.

Tingling: This sensation generally indicates some inflammation. You must use your own immediate perception to decide whether it is chronic, sub acute or acute. The intensity of the tingling may provide a clue. Very intense tingling, sometimes extending up to the shoulders, often signals some acute, severe inflammation. If you are a physician or holistic practitioner of natural therapeutics, you should have the erythrocyte sediment rate (ESR) determined in order to gain more clarity. If you are not qualified to conduct such tests, you should refer your client to another medical practitioner. Reiki is a powerful support tool in such cases, and is effective on its own in less severe cases.

Coldness: This could be caused by an old energy block which dampens the vitality of the organism as it is removed from the flow of ongoing processes. These areas sometimes need a great deal of attention in order to release such energy blocks. A willingness in your client to face old pain or deep forgotten memories may be necessary to release these probably colder areas. Whole body treatment is recommended in addition to extra attention on the cold spot. There is often great potential for growth when this kind of blockage is released. Deep inner work will usually be required before it can unfold.

Heat: If you feel heat in your hands, you may interpret this as a sign that vitality is needed and welcome. The sensations can be anything between warmth and "boiling" heat (although not unpleasant). A tired but vital organism takes in the force it needs. If the sensations of heat are perceptible on the whole body of your client, it does not matter on which area of his body you allow Reiki energy to flow, as life energy automatically flows to the needy areas without much resistance. In such cases reactions that are difficult to deal with rarely arise.

Strong magnetic attraction: This sensation probably infers that Reiki energy is urgently needed in this area and readily accepted. When the feeling of a strong magnetic pull ceases, wait for a while to find out whether another sensation follows. You may then perceive a different vibration. If this is not the case, proceed with the next position.

Energy "pushing" you away: Here we probably have an old, deeply rooted blockage which impedes the vitality and the life energy it needs. Such blocks are usually connected with the vital processes of the body in some form. Clarify whether your client is ready to embark on a process of gaining greater awareness and consciousness. If so, use supporting measures such as the blockage-releasing techniques of the mental method of Second Degree Reiki followed by affirmations or other appropriate means to prepare the individual for opening up. Here you should be aware of your client's anxieties and allow adequate time for the process to unfold.

Flowing: This feeling in your hands suggests that life-force energy is already flowing and welcoming the additional vital impulses, resulting in a higher vibrational frequency of the entire system. Every Reiki session is felt as a merging into love and security. A most agreeable occasion for experiencing gentle growth.

Sharp pain: This may be a symptom of an energy build-up in the process of dissolving. The released energy rises into consciousness and is integrated by the surrounding energy system. The confrontation with parts that were previously repressed is often stressful or painful. In this case, you should not complete the Reiki session too early, but rather treat the whole body. Do not forget the support required afterwards and provide assistance to facilitate integration of the released energy.

Dull pain: This sensation may draw your attention to an old build-up which is still in the pre-conscious state but—as the reaction shows—ready for release. Wherever this sensation is observed, you will have to infuse the area with Reiki energy more often until the hardened structure is completely dissolved. Whole body treatment is not absolutely necessary, but it could speed up release of the blockage. Carefully observe the process. When the build-up starts to release you can then shift your focus to Reiki whole body treatment.

Pain twinges: An energy build-up ready for release, but not yet integrated by the surrounding energy system. Additional, regular Reiki work is required which should also definitely include the rest of the body.

There are also other methods for perceiving energy states through the hands, such as the possibility of feeling the activity of the chakras (also see Chapter Eight). Have your client stand erect or sit on a stool. Now hold one hand at the front and one hand at the back of the body with the palm turned toward the body on the level of a chakra. Feel into your hands; What are your hands perceiving? Make separate notes on every chakra for the front and the back respectively, and evaluate them according to the criteria described in this and the following chapter. Sometimes it is also worthwhile to include certain minor chakras in this check-up.

It may happen that your client's perceptions are quite different from your own. This should not confuse you. Go by your own feelings to judge if you are acting as the Reiki channel or not. Your feelings are very relevant in this case. Generally speaking it is best to avoid giving your client a detailed account of areas with blockages and their deeper meaning. This only creates confusion and sets the client's mind spinning. If you are trained in counseling you will be able to use your knowledge to the benefit of your client.

Another possibility of locating blockages is the pendulum. In the Appendix you will find the respective pendulum tables for the chakras, the most important organs, and various measures which may accompany a Reiki session, and which will facilitate healing work for both you and your client. If you have no practise using a pendulum, you should spend some time learning and gathering experience before working with the tables. The pendulum is certainly a very useful instrument, but also one that is easily misunderstood. You may also refer to the recommended books on this subject. There are various ways to consult the tables as indicated by the following examples:

- "What is the cause of the health disorder?" (Clarify whether there is more than one cause, as this is also a very real possibility!)
- "On what organs, chakras, #query#meridians or parts of the body should Reiki energy be focused? (Are there additional areas requiring special attention. If so, which ones?)
- What organs, chakras, meridians or parts of the body do not need to be supplied with Reiki energy at present? (Examine whether there are several areas which can be excluded!)
- "Which preparatory measures should be taken?"
- "Which measures are required for aftercare?"
- "Did I make a mistake in using the pendulum on any of the questions?

Your client need not be present while you work on these questions. A photo, a specimen of his handwriting or a good personal impression will do. After every Reiki session you can also go through these questions to assess whether some basic changes have occurred which would necessitate different measures.

If you do not have your tables at hand you may use the pendulum directly over the body. You should be well familiar with the manner in which your pendulum indicates "yes", "no" and "don't know" before assessing the individual areas.

Moreover, in specific Reiki work you may use the pendulum to guide you to that area of the body which has the greatest need for Reiki at the moment. Your client should lie in front of you, while you ask the following: "On which area of the body will Reiki have the greatest effect now?" Allow your pendulum to guide you. It will indicate the direction and stop above the respective area or make an "affirmative pattern". Clarify pendulum response patterns beforehand.

But you may also work "mentally", that is without contact and without pendulum dowsing tables. In doing so, you should check each chakra, organ or meridian. Afterwards direct Reiki to those areas which the pendulum affirmed.

As is true for all the other "systems of diagnosis" presented here, pendulum dowsing is only important if you assume that your Reiki work with a certain client is likely to meet with difficulties or if you want to find the areas which most need to receive Reiki energy. The methods are all well-tested in practise and have proved to be very effective. Also keep in mind that as a Reiki channel you are simply that—a channel—and that the effects of treatment is determined by God in the final instance. This, however, is no excuse for lack of competence .

If you feel the need to gain further insight into the significance and course of prolonged Reiki treatment, you could draw on one of the many traditional oracle systems. The Tarot (fortune-telling cards based on the cabalistic teachings), runes (an ancient Germanic symbolic system for representing basic universal energy patterns) or the I Ching (an ancient, over 4000-year-old Chines oracle system exhibiting almost mathematical precision) may provide invaluable assistance. You should be well acquainted with any of these systems before addressing any serious questions, as errors of judgment could have far-reaching consequences.

I prefer working with the I Ching and have developed, by means of a classical translation, a system for assessing subtle conditions. Its scope includes the chakras, the meridians and organs. Inner processes of transformation may also be made more conscious with a system using the I Ching. An adequate presentation of this extensive subject would require a book of its own. I currently teach the practical application of this system in special seminars.

Summary
Various methods for tracing disturbances in the subtle energy system

Main areas of Reiki treatment and areas to be avoided can be traced through:
- Pendulum dowsing (with tables, directly or mental)
- the use of the I Ching or other oracle systems you are very familiar with.

Blockages can be assessed by:
- Sensations in the hands
- Oracle work
- Knowledge of bioenergetic connections

The hidden causes of health disorders can be elucidated through:
- Oracle work
- Therapeutic counseling (provided you have adequate training in client-centered therapy)

However, it is not necessary that the methods presented in this chapter are continuously applied. They are primarily intended for difficult cases. If you use them frequently, your intuition will continue to flourish and the more "technical" crutches will gradually become superfluous. Take your responsibility seriously and reassess the accuracy of your judgment repeatedly.

Chapter Eight

Chakra Work with Reiki

The chakras are subtle energy centers in the human being. The term chakra is of an Indian, or more precisely a Sanskrit origin, and means, among other things, "circle" or "wheel". The chakras have been known in traditional Asian medicine for thousands of years and are used for diagnosis as well as for treating disorders on the physical, emotional and mental levels. They have a variety of functions. On the one hand they are the subtle counterpart of the material organs or groups of organs associated with them. On the other hand they determine how our existence develops on the different planes of being, thus reflecting our respective state of evolution. The system of the chakras is divided into major and minor chakras. These in turn are connected with the meridians and reflex zones known in acupuncture. Moreover, the chakras are embedded in a more highly developed system. As far as I know the only exact descriptions of these planes are given in Indian and Polynesian mysticism. I believe it is important to discuss their significance with reference to Reiki work on chakras, because certain problems cannot be eliminated merely through the respective chakras that are involved. The chakras have an important function, as they link the high subtle planes to the lower and material levels. If a blockage is released, for instance, on the karmic level with the respective chakras not fully functioning, this released energy will not become fully effective on the material level. This kind of dysfunction is actually found rather frequently in subtle treatments. How many times does one hear people sigh to the effect of "I've already done so much for my spiritual development and yet I'm still suffering from this physical disorder which simply won't disappear!"

On the other hand, "repairing" a chakra is not always sufficient for healing and improving your life circumstances. This kind of treatment necessarily remains superficial if ultimately there are unreleased complexes on the karmic levels hidden beneath.

The following hierarchy comprising five levels may serve as a basic blueprint of the energy system we are dealing with:

Material Pole

▽　　　　　▽

Area I: Organs (e.g. liver), nerves (e.g. trigeminus)

Area II: Meridians (e.g. kidney meridian)

Area III: Minor chakras (e.g. energy center in the hands), major chakras (e.g. solar plexus)

Area IV: Individual karmic level (e.g. individual guilt complexes and formations derived from previous incarnations)

Area V: Social karmic level (e.g. group-related and socially-related formations and guilt complexes (catchword: "collective guilt")

△　　　　　△

Ideal Pole

This arrangement is very useful for the assessment and treatment of physical disorders. With the help of the pendulum, by careful questioning of the client or working with an oracle you are familiar with you will be able to ascertain on which energetic level the blockage discovered during treatment has its roots, and then specifically impact it through Reiki. This saves a lot of time which would otherwise have to be spent on superficial or deep energy work. The more organic and acute a disorder, the more quickly Reiki will affect it. Blockages on the karmic level, i.e. individual and group karma, can only be released through regular and prolonged Reiki whole body treatment in conjunction with additional therapeutic measures. Reiki reaches all the blocks on all levels, but in the areas IV and V it is imperative to act out the energies that became "stuck" there and experience them in some way. Reiki provides the stimulus, arouses curiosity and gives strength. But it does not relieve you of the responsibility of actually experiencing the forces taking effect in your life.

Here are some suggestions of how you can use Reiki to harmonize disorders on the following levels:

- Area I: Local application of the Reiki force, in this case channelling it into the affected organs and their respective reflex zones
- Area II: Use Reiki along the meridians and main organs
- Area III: Chakra balancing; specific chakra and Reiki work with minor and major chakras
- Area IV: Whole body treatment; mental treatment with Second Degree Reiki: supplementary work with the respective major chakras
- Area V: Whole body treatment; mental treatment with Second Degree Reiki; supplementary work with the respective major chakras

This list is not to be understood as simple "directions for use", rathermore the examples have been provided to stimulate further thought. If you feel inclined to use other methods, please do so. Reiki is extremely effective, but—as everything else here on earth—not a panacea relieving everyone in every situation of every disease.

Practical Examples of Disorders on Different Plans;

The typical "accident in the kitchen", a finger injured by a knife while cleaning vegetables, does not require Reiki treatment of the first, second and third chakra; this kind of treatment will only be necessary in case of major accidents of this type. To stop minor bleeding and prevent complications it will suffice to keep your hand at some distance above the wound to stop minor bleeding and prevent complications. If a disorder penetrates deeper, affecting the nerves, it has to be balanced with Reiki energy there as well, after having treated the wound immediately. To give an example; you are so nervous and unconcentrated that you cut your finger. In this case, after treating the wound, it is advisable to balance the two halves of the brain and harmonize the solar plexus with Reiki, to help eliminate the causes of the injury.

An area of the chakras is probably affected if someone constantly cuts himself or suffers repeated injuries, without organic problems (such as bad sight) explaining this tendency. If someone is prone to accidents, a disorder in the first chakra might be the cause. This person unconsciously allows damage to be caused to his person. His "will to live" is, for some reason, not strong enough to prevent constant accidents. In this case the pelvic region should be treated with Reiki and, as the therapist, you might try to find the cause of this tendency together with your client so that it can be dissolved along with specific Reiki work.

If feelings of guilt are the cause of the tendency for self-injury, the karmic areas also have to be included in treatment. To this end you should apply whole body treatment and mental treatment of Second Degree Reiki.

Of course you may embark on effective Reiki treatment without previous analysis of the problem, but you will probably have to wait longer for the results in this case. Certain processes may be delayed, as without a clear analysis the right starting-point could be missing, which otherwise might make the subconscious of your client curious and thus more receptive to Reiki.

The interconnections described in this chapter will assist you in arriving at a first assessment of the conditions embodied by your client on his subtle level. If you are interested in further information, you should attend seminars on chakras, anatomy, and acupuncture/acupressure and/or study relevant literature. Please refer to the bibliography in the Appendix for a list of recommended titles.

There are a large number of books on chakras that are worth reading. This great variety of literature on offer may also confuse beginners. It may be difficult to find your way through the many different classifications and systems. Classical Hindu yoga defines six energy centers, Tibetan Buddhist yoga five or six, and Taoist yoga seven. And even that is not the whole picture, for contemporary teachers often even speak of nine major energy centers, since the number nine corresponds to the nine planets. The most advanced systems today describe up to twelve energy centers.

There is not only disagreement with regard to number, as some systems even differentiate between the root and sexual chakras, while others place these two chakras together.

The sexual chakra is often also called spleen chakra and located in the region of the spleen. Some teachers say that the third chakra is below the navel, while others place it near the solar plexus. This list of inconsistencies could easily be continued, but I believe the challenges of the various chakra doctrines have become obvious. When I began studying the subtle processes in my body I felt just as confused as you probably are feeling right now. How to unravel the tangle?

It is quite simple; all of the systems are correct.

Are you still confused? I will attempt to explain what I mean. You may recall the diagram of the hierarchy of the energy system of man; it extends from the material pole on one side to the #query#ideal pole on the other side.

"Material" also means: made of matter; tangible and definable; can be measured and weighed; inert; analytically comprehensible; objectively perceptible; it is the formed and shaped pole (yin).

"Ideal" also means: energetic; intangible; indefinable; fleeting, flowing and subtle; synergistically comprehensible; timeless; subjectively perceptible; without shape and form (yang).

There can be no doubt that the chakras exist. It is possible to prove their existence indirectly with the aid of high-tech electronics, while clairvoyants are able to draw conclusions from their direct perception of the chakras that can be confirmed by other means. Anyone can learn to work successfully with the chakras. Inevitably, different individuals will obtain different results (as is the case with experts in any other field), thereby defining diverging chakra locations and functions.

This is all the more comprehensible if we consider that in qualitative terms chakras belong to the "ideal pole" of existence, which by nature is more "unformed" or "shapeless".

This implies that the location and function of these important energy centers essentially depends on the subjective viewpoint of the observer and that they cannot be fully defined by the "material" aspects of their condition.

Conditions and circumstances such as culture, generally accepted ideas, race, individual karma, priorities of development of the individual and his social group with all its traditions determine the way a human being views his mental and spiritual structure and its manifold functions. It is therefore inevitable that the chakra systems of the Eskimos, Jews, Chinese, Christians and Indians differ from each other on many points. But they nevertheless "work" in each of their different social environments. In every culture there are mystical practices and ways of self-realization to help human beings find their inner core and come to terms with their environment.

But this implies that if you are firmly convinced that you have nine (or three or even seven) chakras and that you find the means to work with these centers you are able to perceive and define in some detail that your chakra work will indeed produce the desired success. This is truly wonderful. But perhaps you've already guessed that there is a catch somewhere; you cannot arbitrarily define your chakras yourself, because they were pre-programmed and are part of your life's plan. So if you had intended to tailor your favorite system, consisting of "64 chakras" and work with it, you are not likely to have any great success in this life. Certain ideas of your inner and outer world have already been established through all the social and traditional connections in which you were born and raised.

How can you put this knowledge that even the chakras are relative to use?

First of all, this view will spare you long considerations and disputes on the correctness of certain systems. There is no need for you to get involved in heated discussions on various authors' opinions, and historical or scientific proofs of different systems. All you have to do is listen and feel inside yourself, and perceive which system suits you best. Then you are ready to embark on your practical work.

Once again proceed step by step; first feel inside yourself to find out which chakra system you perceive within yourself. Once you have discovered that you will know in which framework you have to work, that is, which chakras you will include in your work. Then you are able to start to practice and begin to fill your personal framework with knowledge and experiences. If you have practiced with your own energy system for some time, you will be able to easily verify whether it exists in the form you visualize or whether you have fooled yourself for some reason. Sometimes we like to find a certain system which does not correspond to our actual subjective reality. In this case, Taoist yoga or Chi Kung practices can help us gain the required clarity.

It is very useful for your own work to get to know a self-contained, complete system. If you do that, you will not be forced "to reinvent the wheel". You will have an overview of the best possibilities and interconnections which will help you work with the system which suits you best.

To this end I would now like to present my system. It is as good as any other, but for the time being it offers you the advantage of my own personal experience. As I am very familiar with it I can give you many practical hints.

In addition, as many subtle realities are (as already mentioned above) similar for most people with a common tradition, you will probably be able to work successfully with my system. If you aren't, consider the above mentioned variations and try to understand the system that most suits you. If you have understood just one of the more complex chakra systems, you will have little difficulty in grasping the others and working with them.

Before I discuss any details, please fill out the following questionnaire: For every term on the left side, please note on the right side—without thinking too much—the first three words that come to your mind in their context. This method of association provides you with an initial practical acquaintance with the functions of the chakras and your attitude toward them. In order to do specific work on your chakras with Reiki or any other suitable method, it is essential that you find out which of your chakras are in harmony and those you feel uncomfortable with. You must know which parts you can accept lovingly and which you do not. In this way you are better able to recognize your own limitations and attend to the development of your clients with greater care and awareness. It is only when you are aware of your own issues that you can properly assess the difficulties that may arise during Reiki work, and decide which supporting measures you should take, and what other measures and areas you should exclude.

Chakragram for the Earth Realm

Root Chakra

Life:

Death:

Struggle:

Work:

Child:

Possession:

Earth:

Race:

Sexual Chakra

Touch:

Closeness:

Woman:

Man:

Pleasure:

Consciousness:

Water:

Mother:

Chakragram for the Human Realm

Solar Plexus Chakra

Power:

Personality:

Ego:

Possession:

Fear:

Envy:

Beauty:

Father:

Pride:

Heart Chakra

Love:

Live and let live:

Light:

Healing:

Life:

Union:

Darkness:

Family:

Openness:

Chakragram for the Realm of Heaven

Throat Chakra

Discussion:

Singing:

Voice:

Expressiveness:

Resonance:

Attitude:

Truth:

Public:

Spectator:

Actor:

Audience:

Forehead Chakra

Intuition:

Goal:

Faithfulness:

Intellect:

Knowledge:

Analysis:

Synthesis:

Trust:

Nature:

The terms I have presented in this questionnaire refer to aspects of existence closely connected with the chakras, while the associations you note down reflect your present attitude towards the experiences possible in these realms. They do not provide a complete picture, however, and this is an important reservation to bear in mind. To begin with you should clarify whether the chosen term has a "positive" or a "negative" association for you. For further evaluation you may add a "+" for any association judged positive by feeling, and a "–" for any that is felt to be negative. There is no neutral ground here. In most cases any such neutral ground is a white lie, a mask meant to conceal your attitude, because for some reason you fear your judgment could reveal something you do not wish to see. At the end you should add up the assessments (the "+" and "–" signs) for each of the chakragrams individually.

This short exercise in self-assessment shows you to what extent you are able to accept yourself in the various realms of existence, corresponding to the chakras. A plus sign means "accepted at present", a minus sign "rejected at present ". If you have noted positive assessments everywhere, it probably shows that you have either told yourself a pack of lies, or that in these realms you are presently ready to let reality touch you without any restriction—just as it happens to be. So there will be only minor or no blockages in the plus sign areas. There are no significant obstacles to your self-realization here.

After having done this exercise several times carefully and honestly at intervals of a few weeks, and given yourself much Reiki energy during this period through self-treatments, you will observe changes in your assessments. You are already fully engaged in chakra work with Reiki!

Using the same method you may observe the conditions and processes and development of your Reiki clients. Here a questionnaire may not always be advisable, as many people dislike the feeling of taking an examination. Taking into account such fears, it is better to observe the emphasis and value attributed to terms and aspects which can be assigned to the various chakras during the course of talks with the client. In doing so, do not forget that your glasses too are "colored", and respect the particular characteristics of your client who is your partner in the joint healing process. Otherwise your so-called "awareness" will degenerate into mere prejudice and the trusting openness of the therapeutic relationship will turn into a power game along the lines of, "Now, who is really conscious here and a little more advanced on the path?".

The Opening of the Chakras

If you can accept your chakras in all the realms and live out their energies with pleasure, you are very close to so-called enlightenment and thus in closer contact with the Universal Spirit which takes everything as it is—loving everything and containing everything; not in the limited human sense, but in an all-encompassing manner—for the Universal Spirit or God is unlimited Love.

Terms such as "enlightenment", "God", "Christ energy" refer to the unconditional acceptance of the world. Thus Jesus accepted his disciple Peter as an apostle and friend, although the latter betrayed him three times in the hour of trial.

Now, what does this imply in terms of chakra teaching and Reiki?

The much-acclaimed "opening of the chakras" means that after its completion we are able to accept unconditionally and lovingly all the realms reflected in them. This opening of the chakras is the precondition for the harmonious integration of the awakened kundalini energy into the subtle energy system of an individual.

If the chakras have not been opened at all or insufficiently, the sudden awakening of kundalini energy can bring about a catastrophe in the literal sense of the word. That would be like forcing the water from a fire hydrant through a garden hose. What do you think would happen to the hose?

The chakras can be opened harmoniously with Reiki energy so that the subtle energy system is prepared for using the kundalini in a constructive manner. But before the opening or purification can take place, damaged chakras must be repaired and reconnected to the inner energy system.

During these processes it will inevitably happen that feelings of guilt and fixations (preconceived, stereotyped ideas of how the world should be) will emerge to consciousness. Their dissolution is an indispensable precondition for the opening of the chakras, because a great deal of the energy which we need for the opening and natural function of the energy centers is "frozen" in such complexes.

You may of course accomplish the major part of this work just by using Reiki energy without any knowledge of the chakras. If you are aware of the obstacles you may be facing, the healing process will run a more rapid and yet deeper course.

As you know, Reiki is "drawn in" by the individual receiving treatment. If there are unconscious blocks against those vital changes, little may happen at the beginning.. Assuming that your client really wishes to initiate the healing process in spite of existing blockages, you will be able to create the required conditions through specific

Reiki work and the other methods presented in this book. Few blockages are so deep as to prevent curiosity and the joy of life inherent to the subconscious from awakening. Once this has been carried out, Reiki will flow and stimulate self-healing of the body on all levels.

If a being wants to grow toward higher awareness and a greater capacity for love, he is free to do whatever will help him achieve this kind of freedom, provided of course that others are not harmed against their will. I am well aware of the implications of this statement which are not to be taken lightly. Nature, however, is a good example of how this principle works.

Now let us shift to the functions of the individual chakras: I locate the root chakra very low in the trunk, between the legs, whereas in my system the sexual chakra is found right above the mons veneris (pubic bone). I will discuss these two centers together, because they directly complement each other and both belong to the "earth" realm.

This classification needs a brief explanation. I work with six major chakras (there is another major chakra to be added) and ten important minor chakras. Although there are many more, these ten are quite sufficient in most cases. I use the following terms for the six major chakras:

First chakra	=	root chakra
Second chakra	=	sexual chakra
Third chakra	=	personality chakra
Fourth chakra	=	heart chakra
Fifth chakra	=	expressive chakra
Sixth chakra	=	knowledge chakra

The 10 minor chakras are located as follows:
- Two minor chakras in both palms (they control contact with the environment and the transfer of life energy; on an energy level, they are connected with the kidneys and with the second, third, and fourth major chakras.

- Two minor chakras in the arches of both feet (they control contact with the earth, reception of energy (grounding) and the delivery of "subtle garbage" back to earth; on an energy level, they are connected with liver and gall bladder, with the first and third major chakras and with the aura).
- Two minor chakras just below both shoulders (they control our way of handling responsibility; on an energy level, they are connected with the third and fifth major chakras)

- Two minor chakras in the knee joints (they control the ability to teach and learn as well as flexibility; moreover, the faculty of creating varying energy potentials and gradients which make teaching and learning possible in the first place; furthermore, pride and feelings of inferiority; on an energy level, they are connected with the fifth and sixth major chakras)

- Two minor chakras in the elbow joints (they control our ability to give and accept and our power of self-assertion; energetically, they are connected with the lungs, the pancreas and the second and third major chakras)

The seventh chakra, also called the crown chakra, will not be dealt with here, on the one hand as in my experience it develops through the purification of the other six energy centers, and on the other hand as the processes taking place on the level of the seventh chakra can only be described inadequately by words or pictures. Basically, the seventh chakra can only be understood by direct experience.

I divide the six chakras listed above into three groups; the groups of "earth", "human" and "heaven". Every group includes two chakras, with one of them reflecting and structuring the yang aspect of power (idea) on its level of being and the other the yin aspect of capacity for relationship (experience).

First group = the "earth" plane of existence; its yang aspect of power is in the root center and its yin aspect of capacity for relationship in the sexual center. The first group of the "earth" plane of existence is the basic condition of our existence as beings incarnate in the material realm. It consists of the first and second chakras.

Second group = the "human" plane of existence; its yang aspect of power is in the solar plexus chakra and its yin aspect of capacity for relationship in the heart chakra. The second group of the "human" plane of existence is the basic condition for our humanity. It consists of the third and fourth chakras.

Third group = the "heaven" plane of existence; its yang aspect of power is in the throat center and its yin aspect of capacity for relationship in the forehead center. The third group of the "heaven" plane of existence is the basic condition for our divinity (free development and interaction with the universe). It consists of the fifth and sixth chakras.

The correlation of the chakras with the three realms of existence is no mere theoretical game. This concept has proved to be an extremely useful tool in practise as it presents the essential contents and scope of action of the individual chakras in a concise manner. It enables a quick and reliable overview of the root causes of potential blockages. But here you have to observe carefully on which plane of existence your client is fully alive (and this is also readily ascertained on the physical level) and on which other plane he may tend to be rigid and inflexible. Incidentally, the following crystals are related to the three planes of existence; rock crystal ("earth"), rose quartz ("human being") and amethyst ("heaven"). You will learn more about these in Chapter Twelve.

I have taken my knowledge on the planes of existence from the I Ching which I consider the best textbook on the subject of chakras and the subtle energy system. But utilizing it for this purpose requires some experience and certain keys. Without them the hidden messages cannot be understood. This will be the topic of a later book.

The Chakras in the Earth Realm

Root Chakra

It is the will for survival that expresses itself most strongly in the root center; it is the source of strength for the struggle for survival and for the species-preserving role of sexuality. No living being can develop harmoniously without a properly functioning root chakra. The other energy centers cannot assume the function of this center. It provides the force required in the other centers for contact with the environment and its harmonious utilization for personal growth. Without power nothing works.

The same is true of the will to live (and survive) that is also expressed in this center. That is why in your chakra work with Reiki you should first clarify whether this important energy centers functions sufficiently.

Blockages in the root chakra often result in mental symptoms and attitudes such as extreme pacifism ("I could never kill anyone!"), existential fear ("nobody in his right mind could father children in this world!"), excessive aggression ("shoot those bloody foreigners!"), fear of death ("I'm not willing to take any risks"), problems with order and time planning ("I don't know why I'm always late"), im-

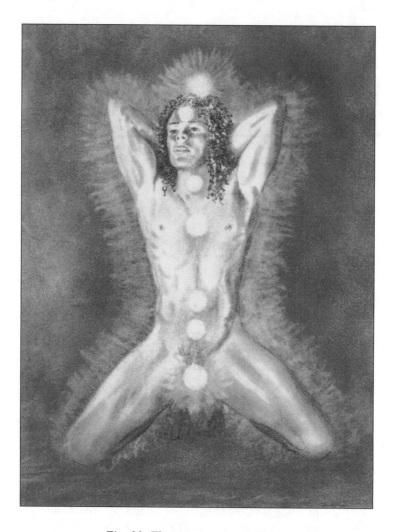

Fig. 30: The seven major chakras
(from bottom to top, chakras 1—7)

patience ("why doesn't this idiot drive off!") and dependence ("I cannot live without him/her/it").

Blockages in the root chakra often produce physical symptoms such as complaints of bones, teeth and spine, diseases affecting the regenerative power, diseases and complaints between the large intestine and the anus.

The maxim for a disordered root chakra; "He doesn't have both feet firmly on the ground".

Sexual Chakra

The sexual center governs our ability to feel the world and, in turn, to be touched by it. According to the hermetic law within, so without, this center also pertains to our capacity for self-perception. Without this perceptive faculty there would be no Eros, no sensuality, no satisfying sexual experience—and no real joy of life either. Coordination of the expression and language of the body (body feeling!), the ability to experience things, sensual pleasure of every kind (enjoyment of culture and art)—we will only be able to experience all of these wonderful dimensions in their full vitality if our sexual chakra pulsates and works without blockages.

Blockages in the sexual center often result in mental symptoms such as fear of physical closeness ("don't touch me!") and disgust with the body ("sexuality is for animals, humans are born for higher things!") But this disgust can also express itself as obsessive washing, cleaning mania etc.), incomprehension ("I don't understand!"), a mind very much centered in reason ("what good are feelings, they won't buy me anything), over-emphasis on spur-of-the-moment feelings ("What's the need for reflection? I just act on instinct. No mind!), rhythmic disorders ("I don't like dancing nor do I dance well!"), ("Why do I always get those menstrual pains?"), ("I prefer working at night!"), isolation ("marriage or partnerships aren't any good for me! No use!"), frigidity, impotence, lacking orgastic reflex ("I don't need sex, I don't see what others get out of it!"), fear of falling ("I would never jump from the ten foot diving-board!"). Whoever is incapable of perceiving his environment adequately or who experiences it as a threat will not be able to protect himself or will pretend to be dead out of fear.

Blockages of the sexual chakra frequently result in physical symptoms such as diseases related to body fluids (blood, lymph, saliva, gall) or the organs processing these liquids (kidney, bladder, lymph glands). In many cases a strong susceptibility to infections is also encountered.

The following statement sums up the condition of a disordered sexual chakra; "He doesn't enjoy life."

If the two chakras of the earth realm are not opened in all their aspects, if they are not lovingly accepted and experienced without limitation in all their functions, then the other chakras will not be able to open completely and will function in a very restricted manner.

The Chakras in the "Human" Realm

The solar plexus or personality chakra is the center of power, the heart chakra being the center of relationship of this realm, governing the personal and social intentions of humans. The endeavors of the ego, that is the self-assertion of your own personality from the solar plexus chakra, represents one pole. Readiness to accept your own ego and that of other living beings in the heart center is the other pole. The will to individuality is what expresses itself in the solar plexus chakra. Its motto is; "It is my will, therefore I am." Consequently, a dysfunction of the solar plexus chakra may manifest rather vehemently in claims to power, dogmatic rigidity, fear of disintegration ("I could lose my individuality, then I'd be dead, just dead and gone"), envy, greed and acquisitiveness.

The solar plexus chakra is extremely important for our path to God, because it is a good starting-point for the dissolution of karma. Here is also the seat of our personal freedom and our feelings of guilt; that is, both our potentially unlimited capacity for growth and our self-imposed limitations. Only when the fears and feelings of guilt as well as the claims to power resulting from them are released that a human being will be able to allow others their freedom, while accepting and loving them at the same time. Thus the way to the opening of the heart is via the solar plexus.

Solar Plexus Chakra

Blockages in the solar plexus chakra often result in mental symptoms and attitudes such as claims to power ("my husband", "my wife", "my child", "my money"), greed ("life isn't worth it, if I don't get a rise, have a lover and drive a new car every year!"), compulsive spending ("I desperately need new clothes!"), status anxiety ("what am I going to do if my boss sacks me, if I don't pass the exam, if my apartment isn't tidy when my friends come and see me") and envy ("now this guy got another new car in front of his garage!").

Blockages in the solar plexus center result in physical symptoms such as stomach complaints, duodenitis, pancreatic dysfunctions, liver and gall complaints, disordered gastric secretions and dysfunctions of the salivary glands.

In cases of an underfunctioning in the solar plexus center, individuals seem nondescript in behavior and appearance.

Overfunctioning usually produces the typical "power-seeker" or "family tyrant". The following line sums up the condition of a disordered solar plexus chakra; "He's attached to the world with every fiber of his being."

Heart Chakra

If the heart chakra is balanced, it enables us to accept the world, ourselves and other persons as they are. If your own personality has been formed in the solar plexus, then the heart chakra is the place for accepting this self-created structure of "personality" with all its rough edges, merits and mistakes, and learning to love it.

The best expression for this task is the commandment "Thou shalt love thy neighbor as thyself." If I do not accept myself and constantly experience inner discord within myself just because I do not live up to my ideal image of myself, because I don't look like Marilyn Monroe or Clark Gable, and I can't sing like Placido Domingo or Tanita Tikaram, then I will not be able to meet my fellow humans in a relaxed and loving manner. Instead, I will accuse them of disappointing me once more, of spoiling my day, of being "capitalist pigs" or "plebs". But if I can take my prejudices and beliefs with a relaxed attitude, I will also recognize the unique capabilities in myself as well as in others. Since I am able to regard these capabilities as helpful and useful, I will accept them joyfully.

Reiki also first operates from the heart center. Healing always takes place whenever the sick part is accepted. But the essence of Reiki is love, "joyful acceptance".

Blockages in the heart center frequently result in mental symptoms and attitudes such as imposing conditions on love ("If you don't do what I want you to do, I won't love you either!"), suffocating love ("My dear child, I only want the best for you!"), exaggerated selflessness ("People are here on earth to help others. Just imagine, if everyone just thought of themselves!") and selfishness ("I'm allowed to, you aren't!" "You have to be there in case I need you!")

Blockages in the heart center frequently result in physical symptoms such as heart trouble, dysfunction of the thymus gland, lung diseases as well as disturbed circulation, tension, cramps, spasms, cancer and AIDS.

If there is a an underfunction of the heart chakra, humans by nature tend to be ruthless against themselves and against others. In case of overfunctioning there will be exaggerated tolerance up to the point of self-sacrifice.

The following line sums up the condition of a disordered heart chakra; "I-he-she-it-must ..."

The Chakras in the "Heaven" Realm

Throat Chakra

The chakras belonging to the "heaven" realm represent the heavenly or divine plane. The throat center governs self-expression and also structures bodily posture, language, facial play, and gestures. Its dysfunction can express itself in demagogy and tyranny. The fifth chakra forms the "interface" to the outside world, with its two poles "self-expression of my personality in unison with the universe" (overtone singing, spiritual music) and "self-expression of wild, exaggerated individuality isolated from the wholeness of life" (Heavy Metal, demagogy, black magic). It reflects our internal world and thus also provides us with an environment that suits us in both the material as well as the social sense. Every inner "poor posture" can be recognized by the external posture and shape of the body.

The motto of the throat chakra is "I show what is inside of me". The Greek hero Orpheus was able to make stones and shrubs weep with his singing. He certainly had a well-functioning throat chakra that was charged with energy. Hitler is an excellent negative example of an individual with a highly-powered throat chakra. With his staccato-like voice, cracking in demagogic cadences, he hypnotized millions of people and held them under his spell.

The harmonious development of the throat center is closely connected with the development of heart energy. "If my ability to love is developed and if I have accepted myself, I won't stifle others with my expressiveness, but harmoniously join in the choir of life." J.R.R. Tolkien describes this in the story of creation of "Simarillion".

Blockages in the throat chakra often result in physical symptoms such as hoarseness ("I can't talk for a long time without getting hoarse"). This hoarseness indicates tense muscles and at the same time may also be a sign of fear of coming out of your shell. If someone believes he cannot express himself properly and appropriately, he will somehow curb his ability for self-expression. A sore throat may also be a symptom of fear. Whatever is concealed behind the symptom can be determined by tension existing in other regions of the body. All the tension in the human body is ultimately given its specific shape by the throat chakra. But this tension is not caused by the throat chakra. The throat chakra only structures the expression of blockages existing in the other chakras. Blockages can be reliably diagnosed by means of the pitch, the existence of overtones and deep frequencies, the flexibility of the voice, its force and endurance. Furthermore, we can influence tension in the pelvic region and in the calves in particular via the throat chakra. And a stiff neck should make me think why I prefer to just look "straight ahead" at the moment. Other typical symptoms of blockages in the throat center are disturbances in growth and development, as the throat chakra is closely connected with the growth-regulating thyroid gland. Indeed, our way of growing is also a form of self-expression. Reiki work on the throat center will promote harmonious physical, mental and spiritual growth in children.

There is also a connection with the solar plexus chakra. The polarity there consisted of the tension between power drive and rejection of power; in the throat chakra it amounts to the overdeveloped or undeveloped ability of exercising power over others.

In case of an underfunctioning of the throat chakra (as in an underfunctioning of the solar plexus center) an individual is usually very nondescript or may even be regarded as retarded. He has difficulty communicating, maybe stammer, keeps getting his words muddled and has a pathological aversion to any kind of extroverted behavior. His head is bent down and his chin is inclined to the larynx. If there is hyperactivity, we find the typical "power seeker". The individual is often hoarse, and speaks with a piercing, shrill voice, and might develop into a little (or large) demagogue, debates for the sake of debate, likes dispute, wants to change the world according to his ideas and offers many well-conceived reasons for it. The individual will tend to carry his head inclined upward with his nose "up in the air".

The following line sums up the condition of a disordered throat chakra; "He never strikes the right note."

The forehead chakra is the seat of our intuition. Intuition is often mistaken for feeling, but it is easy to distinguish between intuition and feeling; whatever I respond to with great aversion, strong disgust or fear, and whatever I absolutely crave and have to have—that is feeling. The neutral ground remaining between is intuition. If you wish to develop your intuition, you first have to learn to understand your feelings so that you can really distinguish between these two, which are often mixed perceptions (your intuition activates certain feelings in you).

The forehead center is also called the Third Eye, because in this area behind the forehead there is a region of the brain which is sensitive to light. Science assumes that in earlier stages of evolution an organ for distinguishing day and night was located there that has disappeared in the meantime. This explanation does not make sense to me, because people with a well-functioning forehead chakra will develop clairvoyance, see the aura etc. Moreover, our eyes are perfectly capable of distinguishing day and night. Naturally, this ability by itself does not tell us anything about the development of the other energy centers. You may also become clairvoyant via the "path of power" which only allows limited and temporary function of extrasensory abilities, brought about by systematic overcharging of the forehead chakra. Eventually a state of "burnout" ensues and gone is the dream of those fantastic psi-powers. There are sufficient reports in relevant literature on Russian "psychokinesis-experts" who found themselves in a wheelchair after a few years of great psychokinetic feats.

In every human being there are potential energetic powers in each of his chakras. Their awakening usually takes place harmoniously in accordance with his ability to accept reality as it is, and to live love. But this kind of natural development is no absolute precondition for so-called "supernatural powers". Any person who seeks psychic abilities can develop them with some patience and self-discipline, but he or she won't become a saint and spiritual teacher doing so. (Therefore, be careful when committing yourself to certain disciplines or teachers ...)

I have already mentioned a large number of the blockages to be found in this center. Functions and dysfunctions are very close to each other here. That is why I have described them together in many cases. The Third Eye is meant to show humans their personal path through the "jungle" of life. This usually happens according to the well-known principle of "trial and error"; first you slip on a banana skin, fall down on your backside and then you stop to think how this kind of mishap might be avoided in the future. The right and wrong tack are sometimes hard to distinguish, as everyone has to tackle his lessons in his or her very own unique manner.

Other blockages of the forehead center result in symptoms such as an aimlessness, a life of instability ("I don't know what I live for), alienation from work ("I don't mind whatever I do as long as the pay is good!") and fear of ghosts, apparitions, phantoms and so forth (caused by hyperactivity). Since our rational cognitive faculty is also seated in the forehead chakra as part of universal knowledge, headaches may occur in cases of too intense analytical efforts, brought about by energetic over-charging of a part of this chakra. Reiki energy radiation toward both feet or simultaneously on both sides of the head quickly restores the balance. Our visual faculty too is structured in the forehead center. Therefore, by way of a person's color perception, short—or farsightedness we are also able to diagnose the energy condition of his body. Dysfunctions of basically healthy and strong organs are also connected with the forehead center. Some other typical blockage symptoms are permanent unemployment, constant relocation, continuously changing lovers, dressing according to the latest fashion trends, adoration of idols, fanaticism and similar things.

If there is an underfunction of the forehead chakra, individuals will tend to be a "dull workhorse" (not in the sense of belonging to any particular class!), along with all stereotypes; a beer bottle and TV, no hobbies, no opinion, no interest in anything, no initiative.

If there is hyperactivity the person may have "visions" ("the mad prophet"), want to warn humanity of impending catastrophes, see spirits, is afraid without knowing why (hyperactivity of the Third Eye in conjunction with a simultaneous blockage in the sexual center). On the other hand, a harmonious functioning of the Third Eye always causes some flow of energy from the root chakra (an indication you have found your path). So always remember this link in case of exhaustion, dullness or insufficient regenerative power.

The following line sums up the condition of a disordered forehead chakra: "He does not find his path".

Reiki will gently promote our opening to the experiences and lessons of the different planes of existence (chakras). Regular Reiki sessions enhance the inner readiness which allow us to become involved in the many possibilities of experience on the two planes of existence (material and spiritual). The speed and character of the experiences are different with every person. Basically, chakras should not be treated separately. Each chakra contains aspects of all the other energy centers, and they are all interconnected in several ways. If we take this holographic structure into account by balancing all the chakras with Reiki energy, we will promote harmonious integration of the experiences on the respective planes of existence within each of the chakras. In chakra work and with Reiki, it is wise to set priorities. The following section will illustrate these priorities.

Practical Chakra Work with Reiki

Chakra Balancing

By using Reiki combined with the following technique we are able to harmonize the subtle energy system in a short time. This method is based on polarity energy work but since Reiki is balancing in effect, it is not important to place a particular hand on a particular chakra, as is the case with pure polarity.

The chakras are always balanced from the extremities to the center, so to speak, by placing your hands on the first (root chakra) and sixth (knowledge chakra) energy centers of your client. Wait until you have the same feeling of energy in both hands. If you have difficulty feeling anything, rub your hands; this will help you focus attention on them. After you have balanced the two outer chakras, repeat the same procedure on the second (sexual chakra) and fifth (expressive chakra) energy centers and then the third (personality chakra) and fourth (heart chakra). If considered appropriate, you can also use other combinations for balancing.

After chakra balancing it is advisable to smooth out the aura to distribute the released energy. If you feel too little energy in your hands, hold every position for about three to four minutes. This is sufficient in most cases. You can also take more time for chakra balancing.

I often use this technique before whole body treatment, and also as a preparation for specific Reiki work. This may help a sensitive client to relax and creates deep receptivity for subsequent energy work.

After a session with significant developments you can use chakra balancing to spread the released energy on a deep level and support the body to integrate the contents that have emerged to consciousness. This gives you a good start to the rest of the day. I feel fresh and centered when getting up afterwards.

Chakra balancing with Reiki stimulates the whole subtle system toward a more harmonious development. If regularly applied, it works like a turbocharger on inner growth processes. Excess energy is distributed and life-force energy is supplied. Chakra balancing also opens the chakras gradually and harmoniously. If performed regularly it will do away with acute energetic imbalances. The capacity of each individual chakra is gradually increased in coordination with all the other chakras.

Every morning before getting up you should balance your chakras with Reiki energy. The results are very convincing, and are a real joy to experience.

Specific Chakra Work with Reiki

The chakras can suffer from three possible disorders or "injuries":
- Obvious defects (fissures or malformations)
- Lacking connection with the inner energy system at the source point (at the spine)
- Lacking alignment (inclined position)

Balancing these disorders is easy with Reiki. But it may take a long time for a disordered chakra to function fully again. A brief laying on of hands (and irregularly at that) is of little help.

Obvious defects and incorrect alignments are best treated in the following way; place one hand on the level of the chakras on the front of the body (outlet point) and the other at the back (source point). In the case of the root chakra, place one hand on the pubic bone and the other on the coccyx. You may and should place your hands on the spine. This is not advisable with other Reiki techniques, since the kundalini energy could be prematurely awakened this way. The outlet point of each chakra is the contact point with the outside world (aura), while the source point is the contact point with the internal world (to the main energy channels lateral to the spine, the direct connection between the kundalini and the sixth chakra—the Third Eye).

When Reiki energy is sent through an injured chakra, it will change back to a correct alignment and fissures and dents will be healed. The flow of Universal Life Energy by or through a subtle organ revitalizes it and enables it to resume its natural function.

Partial Reiki treatment is rarely sufficient, because a defect in the chakra will impair the flow of energy, preventing simultaneous harmonization of all of the parts of the energy center. This is important because every part of the chakra is linked to all the others.

Partial healing will be quickly cancelled by disorders in other parts of the energy center.

The application of Second Degree Reiki mental healing in connection with specific chakra work can greatly speed up and deepen the healing process.

After specific Reiki work on chakras, the chakras should be balanced out. This is because the treated chakra now has a new energetic charge and no longer corresponds to the charges of the other chakras, which can rapidly lead to a new imbalance in the energy center that has just been treated. If all the chakras are balanced by means of Reiki energy, this problem will not arise. Afterwards you should finally smooth out the aura in order to get the released energy flowing again. Then the aura can be detoxified more easily.

Lack of connection between a chakra and the inner energy system can be restored by channelling Reiki into the affected chakra on the back of the body. Give the client two to three minutes to absorb the energy at this place and then proceed with the technique as described above. This procedure can be repeated a few times. Here too treatment is completed by chakra balancing and smoothing out the aura. If you have a feeling that the aura should be smoothed out more than three times, repeat the procedure until you feel satisfied with the result.

Chakra Balancing with Three People

This exercise is extremely suitable for treatment sessions in which basic blockades are to be dealt with gently, but it can also be employed as a preparatory step for specific chakra work, as a means of quick relaxation or "just for fun".

The person to be treated lies on his back and places his hands on his solar plexus and his heart center respectively. It is advantageous if the client also has Reiki initiation, but this is not a necessity. The correct placing of his hands is only necessary if he is not an initiate, in which case the left hand should definitely be placed on the heart center and the right on the solar plexus center.

The two people giving treatment sit to his right and left. One of them places his hands on the root and forehead center, the other balances the sexual and throat centers. In this way all the chakras are balanced simultaneously. Due to the restfulness of this method (there is no change in position) deep relaxation is more easily achieved than with whole body treatment. On the other hand, organs for the main part are only acted on indirectly. For this reason this kind of chakra balancing is more appropriate for relaxation, working on chronic blockades, general strengthening and calming. Before and after the session it is helpful to smooth the aura. After this, energy stroking should be performed to connect the harmonized chakras with the earth energy.

Please note: After any deep state of relaxation you should sit up slowly and take your time finding your way back to normal reality.

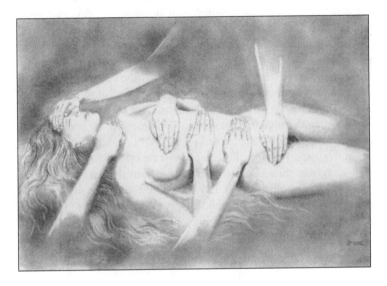

Fig. 31: Chakra balancing with three persons

Specific Reiki Work on Major and Minor Chakras

If there are problems with certain minor chakras, they can generally be favorably influenced by balancing them with the major chakras connected with them or with other major chakras you consider relevant.

If no improvement becomes evident after several sessions (at least ten applied daily or at two-day intervals), the same methods can be applied as above for healing the major chakras. Afterwards the minor chakras have to be harmonized with the respective major chakras, and balancing of the major chakras will be useful at the end.

Successful Reiki work on the chakras requires regular and frequent sessions. The healing and growth processes activated in this way are of a very deep nature, which is why the client should live a calm and harmonious life during the whole period of treatment. It is not possible to "fix" disordered chakras "just casually", even with Reiki. Often the treatment has to be supplemented by homeopathic or psychotherapeutic techniques.

In my experience chakras heal most rapidly if Reiki treatment also integrates naturopathic remedies and psychotherapeutic techniques into one holistic effort. Laymen should neither prescribe medication nor tinker around psychologically in this respect. There are enough specialists for this purpose.

Pendulum dowsing tables for analysing disorders in the energy system are to be found in the Appendix.

Summary
Chakra Work with Reiki

The following questions have to be clarified before and during chakra work with Reiki :

- At which level is the root of the disorder? (A physician or practitioner of natural therapeutics should always be consulted in the case of serious physical or emotional problems.)
- Which major and/or minor chakras are affected?
- How detailed should Reiki treatments be? (Determine type, duration and frequency of treatment.)
- Are other methods to be included in treatment? If so, which? Are you properly qualified? If not, which therapist should be consulted?

If you assume there might be karmic connections or fixations (requiring Reiki on the solar plexus), whole body treatment should be applied along with psychological treatment. It is only when the karmic load with its mental blocks has been dissolved that a deep healing process will be initiated along with personal growth. The result will be quite naturally a higher ability to love and greater awareness.

An explanatory note: By fixations, I mean preconceived notions (dogmas) or judgments which lay down how the world and humans have to be (or not be) so that everything is in a state of order. These kind of blocks often express themselves in rigid moral concepts. In the long run it is impossible to base your life on such ideas. If they deviate from them, while not recognizing the harmfulness of their beliefs, karmic loads will be formed, that is guilt complexes preventing a human being from recognizing and accepting love as the proper foundation of life. Guilt is always linked with fear; it has nothing to do with love, and in fact even excludes it. Since God (Universal Spirit or Mind) is love, imaginary guilt prevents humans from entering into a relationship with God (Love).

Chapter Nine

Reiki and Crystals

Throughout history, stones and crystals have been used for curative treatments, protective spells and initiation ceremonies of all kinds. Their beauty and the light they radiate have become popular again today, at the beginning of the New Age. Many people have adopted the use of crystals to become attuned to the vibrations of the Aquarian Age that we are now entering.

Precious stones can also be of valuable help to us in the application of Reiki. This subject has been dealt with in detail in a new book by Ursula Klinger-Raatz. In this chapter I will be discussing some applications that are easy to perform and yet very effective, and which have evolved out of my study of Reiki and crystals.

Reiki helps to initiate a number of deep inner processes. Fears and hidden parts of the personality requiring integration for the betterment of mental and spiritual growth arise to consciousness. This results in a difficult inner situation; the old ways begin to appear meaningless, but new ways are not yet in sight. Some of the blockages are very stubborn and fear of the contents urging to emerge into consciousness can lead to painful cramping or nightmares. During this process our friends from the realm of minerals can be of valuable help.

According to my experience of Reiki sessions and seminars, three crystals (amethyst, rock crystal and rose quartz) have proven to be especially effective. While their inherent traits are very different, they work well together, and can effectively support Reiki work as well. The following includes suggestions of my own.

Rock crystal illustrates the true quality of light, rose quartz awakens in us the resonance of its vibration of love energy and helps us accept the truth of light, while energetically the amethyst activates the Third Eye and helps point out one's individual path toward realization.

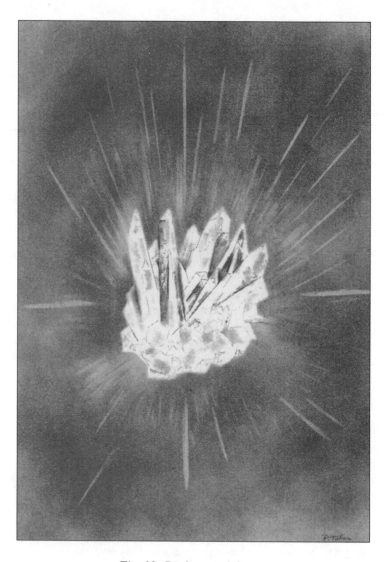

Fig. 32: Rock crystal druse

Rock Crystals

Rock crystal represents the highest stage of evolution in the realm of minerals. No crystals are exactly alike, but they often grow in families with a common base (grouping). The six sides of a crystal are related to the six chakras in humans and its tip corresponds to our center of transformation, the seventh chakra (crown center). At the base it is often cloudy and becomes clear toward the top. Somewhat like humans the crystal grows from out of the gross world towards the subtle world and becomes more and more clear and luminous in the process. Its ability to be transparent and receptive to all vibrations can help humans let go of the blocks which otherwise prevent them from being equally receptive.

In my work I use three different forms of these "light bringers", each of them serving a very specific purpose; a small grouping with two large and one small crystal (diameter at the base about three centimeters, height about six centimeters); a single crystal about ten centimeters long; and two egg-shaped polished crystals about three and a half centimeters in diameter. The sizes are of course approximate. You may choose suitable stones you intuitively feel attracted to, according to the purpose.

In the course of regular treatment with Reiki energy, parts of the Self will rise to consciousness which you may find difficult to accept. At the same time you develop more sensitivity, while becoming more open to new experiences. On the other hand you must learn how to protect yourself when too many or upsetting new experiences overcome you. These learning processes are reflected in your dreams and also in your relationship to your surroundings. Rock crystal can help ensure that you are not overwhelmed by the many changes and the new level of energy that accompany them. Generally speaking, rock crystal helps ease the way through stormy seas.

A small grouping can have a miraculous effect in the case of disturbing dreams. Simply place it at the head of your bed and clean it every two to three days (see details in the Appendix, p. 191).

At home or work you may often come across people who know which of your buttons to push to make you cross, insecure etc., people who drain your energy or constantly have a negative attitude. In this case, carry or wear the crystal somewhere on your person so that it is always with you. It will literally bring light into your daily routine. This work is strenuous for crystals so you need to clean them regularly. If you wish to show appreciation for their work, you can treat them with Reiki.

If you ever feel overwhelmed by some of the new situations life brings to challenge you, and things seem to get beyond your capacity producing a lot of stress, you can practice two variations of Reiki meditation as described in Chapter Eleven. These techniques will help you release anxieties and blocks.

Reiki Meditation
with Rock Crystals

Variation A

Lie on your back, draw up your legs and allow your knees to fall apart. Place the soles of your feet against one other as completely as possible. Finally, place your hands together, as in a gesture of prayer, in front of the heart region while holding in between them a reasonably sized and polished rock crystal. Instead of lying, you can do this meditation in a seated position, leaning against a wall or a chair.

The energy of the crystal is received through the minor chakras in the palms of your hands, entering the entire body via the reflex zones. If you urgently need light, the light bringer will feel very hot after a while. This need not frighten you, as it is quite a normal reaction to the large amount of energy being released. Along with receiving the effects of the crystal, you also channel Reiki as in whole body treatment, via the reflex zones and acupuncture points on your hands. The cleansing, blockage-releasing effect of the rock crystal helps Reiki to flow more easily. During this exercise focus your attention on your hands, feel the energy spread and notice the reactions in your body. If you wish you may also combine this technique with the powerful mantra OM (for more details, see Chapter Eleven).

Variation B

Here you take the same position as above, placing your arms, bent at an angle of about 45 degrees, on the floor. The palms should face upwards. Place a polished, round rock crystal onto the palms of your hands. Feel into your hands. Become aware of the energy moving through your body. Variation B is very good for preparation for whole body treatment and is also very effective as meditation. Instead of lying on your back, you can also do this exercise in a seated position, leaning against a wall or a chair.

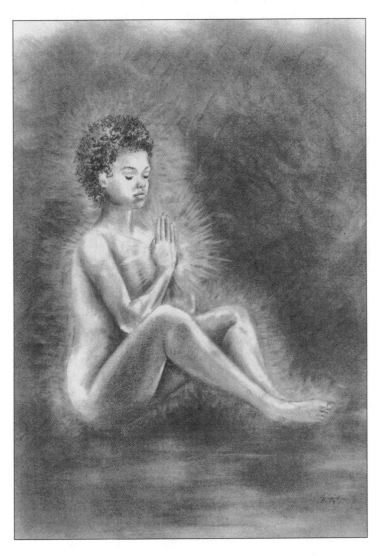

Fig. 33a: Meditation, variant A

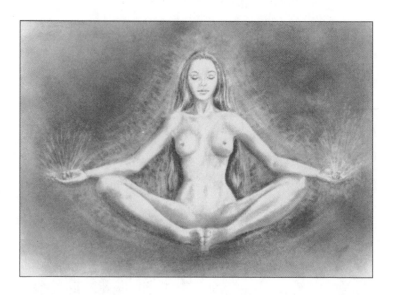

Fig. 33b: Meditation, variant B

These exercises are very intense, which is why the crystals used in them need to be set aside for a few days and cleansed thoroughly. If you feel strong, locally-confined blocks (i.e. tense shoulders or a feeling of fear in the solar plexus), you or your partner can use a long crystal to dissolve them. To do this, move the light bringer above the affected area in a clockwise circle, spiralling upwards and away. You can repeat this procedure several times as required. Sometimes it is advisable to occasionally blow strongly over the blocked zone in order to remove the energy that has been released from the body into the inner aura. Once the blockage has been dissolved or significantly decreased, you can proceed with normal Reiki treatment. Afterward the feet should be treated for at least five minutes and the aura smoothed out.

This method has also proved successful in the case of cramps which can sometimes occur during specific Reiki treatment (see Chapter Six). One client received Reiki in her pelvic region because of menstrual pains. After a short time the cramps increased and were not even to be alleviated with Reiki directly applied to the surrounding areas. (Here the mistake was made of not combining specific Reiki work with whole body treatment!) After using a rock crystal and the technique described above, the cramps ceased very quickly and only appeared rarely and in a much weaker form during subsequent treatment.

Further realms of application for this technique (supported by sub-sequent Reiki work) are:

- Energizing scar tissue (if necessary, have them injected by a practitioner of natural therapeutics or treated homeopathically)
- Specific treatment of organs and lymph nodes
- Healing of damaged chakras (with additional measures as described in Chapters Six and Eight)
- Treatment of wounds (in support of other measures)
- Mental relaxation for people who have difficulty letting go. (during a Reiki session you can put polished rock crystals into your client's hands or place them on the parts of the body that seem to be in need of life energy, but only with the client's consent).

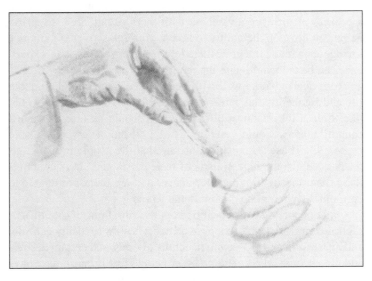

Fig. 34: Blockage release with a rock crystal

Rose Quartz

This crystal belongs to the quartz family. For Reiki work I use polished rose quartz crystals of about four centimeters in diameter. The warm, pink vibration corresponds to the loving quality of the heart chakra. All deep healing is achieved through the energy of this center. The pink light of rose quartz gently reminds the energy bound up in blockages of the love that awaits it, thus raising it to raised to the surface of consciousness. For this reason both rose quartz and rock crystals may be used for the deep release of blockages and for healing physical and emotional problems.

Rose quartz is able to heal experiences of separation and resulting traumas as it often helps them appear in another, more loving context. We experience the most cleansing tears when we allow love into our consciousness. These tears become the visible sign of the experience of "oneness" that suddenly becomes apparent when you are released from the isolation of feeling separate from love. While rock crystals help to illuminate your breakthrough into "oneness" in a process of growing awareness with their vibrations, rose quartz helps you develop the ability to accept your rediscovered parts in a loving manner and integrate them into your personality. This experience can be compared with the return of the prodigal son.

Rose quartz works well with people who often complain about life and frequently indicate—perhaps with a sigh—that they would like to do a lot of things differently ("It would be nice if..., but I cannot!"; "How would I end up if I...!"; "If only everybody would do so...!"). These statements illustrate that the people probably already accept some hidden parts of their personality, but cannot release them through loving acceptance, and are therefore unable to harmoniously integrate them into the whole.

Other people may also benefit from the vibrations of rose quartz, such as dogmatic people, people who reject healthy sexuality or health and aggression and those who reject their bodies and certain desires, and also people who condemn other people just because they have ideas different to their own. If before or during whole body treatment you place a rose quartz on the heart chakra or on chakras representing the special qualities that your client unconsciously rejects, they will help him to accept the respective energy now being released.

If during or after a Reiki session there are feelings of anxiety, place a rose quartz into one or both hands of your client. This will help him to come to terms with and forgive himself. Moreover, assuming Second Degree Reiki mental treatment cannot be applied for some reason after intense specific Reiki work (for example, on the chakras), lay one or several rose quartz crystals onto your client.

If you use rose quartz instead of rock crystals during the forms of meditation described at the beginning of this chapter, they will support you in accepting both yourself and others with all rough edges, faults and weaknesses, so that you do not eat yourself up in helpless anger about the "imperfections of the world". Instead of intoning the mantra OM audibly or silently, you may also work with affirmations such as "I accept myself as I am!", or "God loves me as I am!"

If you feel this exercise might evoke too powerful reactions in you, you could ask a friend you trust to support you during meditation. If you are afraid of this exercise, don't perform it but go to a psychotherapist first to clarify your aversion. The purpose of the exercise is fulfilled the moment you become aware of your aversion to accepting certain parts of yourself. Once you have learned to love yourself, this meditation gives you a wonderful opportunity to bathe in the pink vibrations of love and simply feel good. I often do this exercise after dealing with everyday problems and the chaos within myself and others in order to remind myself of the other, accepting side or reality.

The Amethyst

This violet crystal teaches the lesson of humility. It has the ability to stimulate the Third Eye, thus helping us to recognize and accept our own individual path. With the addition of this stone, my simple system of three crystals is complete, as by using the amethyst we help amplify the vibration which aids the realization of Self within the framework of our universe. Each person has their own personal path; all he needs to do is discover and follow it. However, this is often easier said than done.

The amethyst helps you to harmoniously integrate your new self-awareness into the daily routine of life. During regular Reiki treatment work situations arise again and again that draw your attention to this problem. You are not sure how to integrate your new Self into the world of work, family life and your circle of friends without affecting the new structures you have acquired and without offending people or making them feel insecure.

For Reiki work I use polished amethysts of about four centimeters in diameter. To use the amethyst on yourself, lie down and adopt the

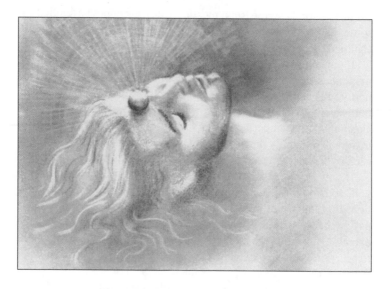

Fig. 35: Meditation with an amethyst

meditation posture in example A as described at the beginning of the chapter. Place an amethyst on your Third Eye and channel the Reiki energy from your left hand into the heart chakra, and from your right hand into your solar plexus chakra.

These positions stimulate your Third Eye and make sure that it is not "overcharged", but rather is balanced by the energies of the heart and solar plexus centers. In other words, this is a method of chakra balancing. When stimulation of the Third Eye enables you to see your path more clearly, fears are often released in the solar plexus. However, since this center itself is being balanced with the loving energy of the heart chakra, this sense of fear acts in an appropriate way as a warning and is unable to tyrannize us. In this way fear is avoided or considerably lessened.

Placed on an organ that has previously been treated for a prolonged period of time with Reiki due to some dysfunction, the amethyst encourages it to resume its proper work within the metabolism. This may be used, for example, as a supporting measure for glandular hyperactivity. Whenever organs you have been working on regain strength, but do not seem to be working appropriately, work with the amethyst as indicated. Furthermore, you may use it for the following symptoms; high blood pressure, angry outbursts, nymphomania and hysterical conditions of all kinds.

During Reiki whole body treatment I often use this "stone of knowledge" locally, or place it on the Third Eye to enable my client to use the supplied life-force energy purposefully, and to prevent anxiety from developing. In the evening after a Reiki session you can place it for about fifteen minutes on the Third Eye, to help you to harmoniously integrate this new vitality into your life.

Summary
Reiki and Crystals

Amethyst (sixth Chakra)
Lesson: Realizing one's own true Self in a universal context
Energy situation: Not properly used
Symptom: Hyperactivity of all kinds; inflammation; high blood pressure; glandular hyperactivity; hysteria

Rose Quartz (fourth Chakra)
Lesson: Accepting
Energy situation: Not accepted as a possibility
Symptom: Resistance of all kinds; cancer, cyst, tension, schizoid symptoms

Rock crystal (second Chakra)
Lesson: Perception
Energy situation: Not realized
Symptom: Underfunctioning of all kinds; poor circulation, glandular underfunctionings; depression.

Chapter Ten

Reiki and Scents

Aromatherapy, or healing with fine scents, has become tremendously popular during the past few years. Ten years ago essential oils were still used almost exclusively for the production of cosmetic perfumes. Their application was more or less limited to beauty care and thus to making us more attractive. Today this situation has changed. Essential oils are now also used for stimulating inner growth processes and for therapeutic purposes.

The scents of essential oils work on an organic level due to the presence of certain typical essences; at the same time they also possess high-potency subtle vibrational patterns that can have a curative influence on the inner energy systems and the aura.

My first experience with the efficacy of these essences occurred during a series of metamorphosis therapy sessions with a friend of mine. She used different perfumed oils to harmonize my chakras before starting a session, which is how I had the idea of using scents at my own Reiki sessions.

I have had some good experience with a system of complementary essences that works very well and which also has the advantage of being easy to grasp. If you would like to use them as a meaningful addition to Reiki, do not think you have to become an expert in aromatherapy first. The system employs the following essential oils; clary sage, patchouli, lavender, lemon verbena and sandalwood.

Clary sage

This very stimulating scent mainly affects the Third Eye. It opens the mind to new vistas of experience by inspiring a new openness and a heightened sensitivity to the sensual pleasures of life. Taking you beyond the level of reason, it evokes the curious, childlike ability to enjoy the world in total wonderment.

For Reiki work I use clary sage to gently open blocked major and minor chakras. Clary sage helps you to sense on a subconscious, pure emotional level the wonder of exploring this new space. It inspires one to drop self-imposed limitations and develop courage to

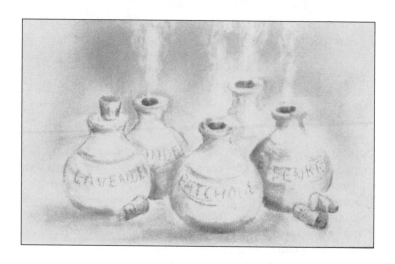

Fig. 36: Various essential oils

face new challenges. Its even, calm quality and its cheerful over-tones instil in us a more lively uninhibited sense of being, and enable us to release locked-up energy.

Patchouli

A sensual, erotic scent. It especially affects the sexual center while increasing sensual perception and zest for life. An increased appreciation of the sensual aspects of life can help you release energy held back in an otherwise blocked pelvic region. Patchouli is more adult than clary sage, because it opens us up to the sensual pleasures on all levels of existence, making us receptive to music, art, sensuality and the joy of experiencing nature. While clary sage inspires an almost naive childlike openness, patchouli knows very well what kind of experiences it seeks to open itself up to; namely sensuous, pleasurable contact with the world and other people.

In Reiki work you may use patchouli to restore the flow of energy in the pelvic region and to help reduce "thick skin" (both in a literal and a symbolic sense), i.e. the self-created obstacles which hold one back from a more sensual encounter with life. This includes the fear of being touched and closeness of all kinds, allergies, skin impurities, and anything else a person may have set up in order not to experience his life on a sensual level.

Patchouli may be used with all major and minor chakras closed to sensual perception to help restore this function. People who do not like patchouli but who would definitely benefit from its effects could try out ylang-ylang, which has similar properties.

Lavender

This noble and reserved scent has proved to be particularly successful with oversensitive people who are easily disturbed, even by a silly joke, and who constantly moan and complain about the rudeness of their fellow humans. Lavender oil also helps people who so deeply hurt and sensitive that they are not even able to voice their anguish. Such symptoms can be traced to a weakened aura. Normally, the aura protects the inner energy system from too strong stimuli, much like an energetic skin. If the aura has fissures or does not flow properly, many impulses can reach the chakras without being filtered and place too much strain on them. Every contact with the environment is then felt more or less as an assault. Often such a weakened person will adopt protective habits to compensate for their heightened sensitivity. They usually only maintain contact with a few selected persons and even then prefer to be alone with these people so that they will not be disturbed by others. They are the type that generally prefer doing their shopping in the store around the corner where they know the owners. On vacation they tend to go to a private family-run bed and breakfast somewhere in the country that they have been familiar with for a long time.

When you decide to treat such an introverted type with Reiki you should try to provide him with the protection he so urgently desires. Here lavender oil can be of valuable help. Find out the most sensitive chakra(s) and apply the oil. The examples I have used here are somewhat exaggerated. They may actually not take on such stereotyped form at a first glance. Nevertheless my description of extreme cases may help you perceive and understand similar conditions on a smaller scale.

Lavender can be very useful during prolonged Reiki work when many new things are being perceived due to the release of blocks and when impressions are generally felt more intensely. When a person is "thin-skinned", he needs protection and peace as he slowly regains confidence in himself and regains contact with his own life-force energy. Lavender can promote this development as it strengthens the energy of the root and solar plexus centers.

This is also true for specific Reiki work and the release of chakra and aura blockages. After a far-reaching release of such blocks the chakras and the aura require protection for a certain period of time. If we fail to provide this, negative reactions may occur very quickly in an even worse form. Blocks and fears are never entirely without purpose. In the past they have had a valuable and important protective function for the person concerned. We must never disregard this fact when they are released.

Lemon verbena

This scent freshens and empowers. Its freshness helps you to become detached from outmoded patterns of behavior and thinking and to accept new, more life enhancing ones. Lemon verbena is indicated if a person has become conscious of his blocks, and all preparations have been made to let go of them for good. The only thing that may be still lacking is the strength or willingness to do so, which creates insecurity. It may seem easier to use a crutch than risk stumbling over legs that function but which unfortunately are still rather weak.

This idea may also be transferred to Reiki work. What it hints at is the importance of making sure that the energy reserves of your client are sufficient for adjusting himself to a new way of life and for releasing his blocks for good if you have restored the function of his organs and energy system in your treatment (which also requires strength). Lemon verbena mainly affects the root chakra, in combination with an opening of the Third Eye. It is therefore advisable to use lemon verbena locally after cleansing and partial opening to strengthen any particular chakra. At the same time, strengthening also provides protection.

Sandalwood

In a certain way this essence evokes the function of the loving, warmhearted mother. Its calm energy pattern creates the sensation of human warmth, acceptance, openness and understanding.

During Reiki treatment you may use this scent to help create a pleasant atmosphere right at the beginning of a session. Your client is more likely to open himself up to Reiki energy and "let go". In other words, sandalwood evokes trust, and this trust must be justified by your behavior. You may also use sandalwood for intense specific Reiki work, as for instance when treating the chakras or loosening muscle armor. Sandalwood oil does not only help establish a feeling of trust, it also facilitates communication. Under the influence of sandalwood, few people will take something the wrong way.

Practical Applications for the Oils

For local application you may mix the oil (pay attention to the quality; synthetic oils can cause illness under certain circumstances) in a ratio of 1:20 with sweet almond oil. If you shake it afterwards ten times, you raise it to a potency as in homeopathy. Its effect will then be even stronger, deeper and at the same time gentler.

Locally, those oils may be used for the treatment of chakras, emotional armor, tension etc. They are also effective when applied to the hand and foot reflex zones.

To use essential oils locally, put a few drops of oil on your middle and index fingers and rub it on the respective area of the body in an anticlockwise direction with gentle, circling movements spiralling inwards towards the end.

You may also use an aroma lamp to fill the consulting room with the scent of the desired essence. For this you put a few drops of the pure essential oil into the bowl which is filled with water. For sandalwood and patchouli you may also use incense sticks, but they have to be of good quality and consist of pure, herbal materials.

If you want to merge your whole day in the vibration of a particular essential oil, simply put a few drops on some cotton wool or a paper handkerchief. Wrap a little more cotton wool or tissue around it and put the scent package into a small bag that you wear round your neck on a silk or leather string (in no case use a chain of any kind of metal!). This indirect method keeps the fragrance and vibration of the essential oil longer in your aura than a perfume applied directly to the skin.

Summary
Reiki and Scents

Clary sage: Awakens the joy of life and the natural curiosity of the "inner child".

Patchouli: Awakens the pleasure of sensuous experience and joy in the perception of the world around you.

Lavender: Suitable for oversensitive people; strengthens the protective function of the aura; creates security by establishing a sense of distance.

Lemon verbena: A powerful tonic; eliminates organic and metal instability; provides the energy to actually use the energy released by treatment.

Sandalwood: The loving, warm-hearted "mother" of the essences; evokes an atmosphere of trust and facilitates communication.

Chapter Eleven

Reiki and Meditation

Meditation in all its forms has been a popular means of self-discovery ever since ancient times. Through different methods of contemplation the student attempts to realize his Self, that is, to consciously experience his true being. Success in meditation practise is essentially linked to two principles; letting go and non-doing, with non-doing making letting go possible. Only when you are not continuously active in some form can you free your consciousness of its contents and thus let go of your "hold" on reality. At the same time letting go is an indispensable condition for non-doing; you have first to let go of compulsive action caused by fear for non-action to develop in free space. Sounds complicated, doesn't it? How can the problem be solved? In other words, how can you meditate successfully?

Quite simply, with joyful, loving acceptance. If you observe during meditation that your mind is already busy tidying up your apartment, for example, don't dwell on these thoughts or on the idea that they are out of place and disturbing. You are sitting or lying down and everything is OK. Realize that you are involved in the necessities of day-to-day life and that you cannot suddenly shake off whatever it is that is otherwise important to you. Don't punish yourself if your attention wavers. Drop your claims to power by consciously perceiving that you have them. Of course you want to remain in control of your life. Try to understand your claims to power by becoming aware of the fears that cause these claims; the fear of life turning into a catastrophe if you don't keep everything under control; the fear of your husband or wife not loving you any more or even leaving you if you don't take care of this or that, not to mention all the other horrid ideas resulting from the delusion of "being separate" from the world that each of us has.

Is your back hurting from sitting? In that case perceive the pain which shows you that your muscles are holding back the energy to their absolute limits. Do you want to open your eyes, become aware of the world again and continue your activities where you left off? In that case look at your restlessness and follow it to its physical or inner roots. Don't suppress it. Rather give it the attention it deserves because it is also part of you.

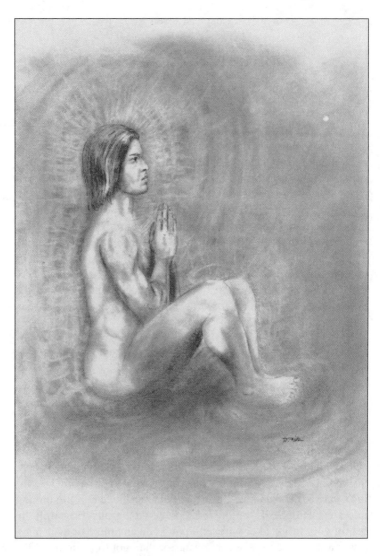

Fig. 37: Reiki meditation—exercise I

Or is it that you don't want to pay attention to yourself right now? It is more important to look after your cats, entertain your wife or your husband? Follow your motives to the fears that are their root. That is all you have to do. If you do this, you have already meditated seriously for quite some time!

Reiki can effectively support the process of concentration on the Self and subsequent letting go with the deep relaxation that this entails. You can hardly avoid meditating when you perceive the flow of energy and establish calm contact with your body, particularly in view of the effect of Reiki as such.

You just have to allow some time for meditation. If parts of your Self that frighten you enter your field of consciousness, Reiki energy will help you to gradually and lovingly accept them and to integrate their precious energy into your whole being. It is only after this has taken place that the process that leads from analysis (observer—object of observation) to synthesis (integration through conscious, loving acceptance without logical reasoning) can be said to be complete.

In the following I have compiled some meditation exercises that are especially suited for combination with Reiki.

Reiki Meditation—Exercise I

Lie down on your back, draw up your legs and let your knees drop to both sides. Press the soles of your feet together so that they touch as completely as possible. Now join your palms in a gesture of prayer in front of the heart region. You may also do this meditation exercise leaning against a wall or an armchair in a sitting position if you prefer (see Figure "Reiki meditation—Exercise I")

What exactly happens during this exercise?

By joining the minor chakras in your hands and feet you complete your energy circuit. Reiki energy can now be set in motion via the contact of your hand chakras with the reflex points to all areas that are energetically under-supplied. It now starts to flow to an ever-increasing degree through your crown chakra into your body. From there Reiki is drawn down toward the solar plexus and then directed to your hand chakras via the heart center, spreading via the meridian system and the reflex zones to all areas of your body requiring additional life energy.

Moreover, Reiki also flows directly through your arms into your body. To do this, Reiki energy first has to release all the blockages it meets on its path or at least create a passage through them, as other-

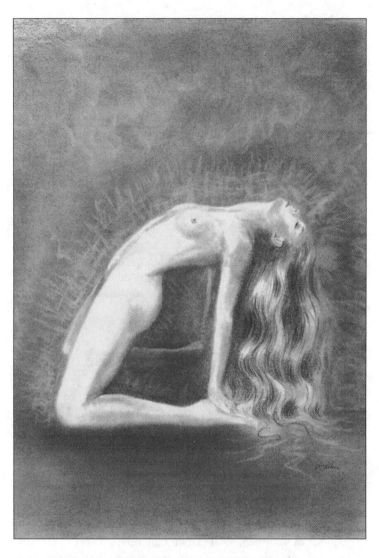

Fig. 38: Reiki meditation—exercise II

wise it will not be able to really flow through you. If you do this meditation exercise regularly, you will feel the energy moving up into your arms more and more, causing a pleasant, tingling and flowing sensation wherever it reaches.

In this way your attention gets increasingly focused on your body and your true Self. Along with this process, Reiki releases blockages, filling them with love and warmth and giving you a feeling of wholeness; yes, you are accepted.

This exercise, which is already powerful enough in itself, may be further extended by simultaneously intoning the mantra OM. This word of power is of Sanskrit origin and means "thus it is!". By intoning OM, you create its vibration in your body, making your body the sounding board of its energy. The "o" is felt as a vibration in the direction of the Third Eye. Jointly, the two sounds of OM enable you to feel the poles of your Self. The mantra makes you conscious of your connection to heaven and earth, the forces of yin and yang. This physical awareness helps you to accept yourself to a greater degree. You are able to feel yourself and can thus direct your attention, your own energy and Reiki energy into these two poles within your Self. This flow of your life energy to your poles quite naturally extends the limits of self-perception, limits that you may not previously have allowed yourself to cross. Your possibilities for self-expression expand; you open up to more energy and greater zest for life.

During the exercise you should breathe from your stomach. At first do this exercise for three minutes. Once you get used to it, increase the duration in small steps. In Tibet they say that a human being may realize the state of oneness with the universe by continuous chanting of the mantra OM.

Reiki Meditation—Exercise II

This exercise directs your attention to your state of groundedness and makes you distinctly aware of the power you have. At the same time the flow of Reiki strengthens your root chakra, removes blockages in the region of the feet, legs and pelvis and strengthens the function and energetic properties of your aura. Moreover, all regions of the body are reached and harmonized via the meridians and foot reflex zones. That is why this method is also very much recommended if there is a tendency for headache and general energy blockages in the upper half of the body.

Kneel down on your haunches on a soft, though not too pliable surface with your legs spread a little wider than your shoulders. Now place the palms of your hands on the soles of your feet and lean backwards until you touch the floor with your back. This exercise is equally effective if you practice with an erect back. It is important to cover your big toes and the center of your metatarsal arch with your hands (see the illustration). At the beginning stay in this position for about five minutes and increase the duration of the exercise gradually.

Here's another variation of this exercise; kneeling in an erect position stretch your pelvis forward and hands and let your head hand backwards with your hands touching the soles of your feet (see Figure 38). This exercise is wonderfully effective for healing your chakras, but it will cause a lot of strain at first. It is best to start for only half a minute and gradually increase the duration.

After meditation it is advisable to bend forward—still on your knees until the upper part of your body and your face are on the floor with your arms parallel to your body. Maintain this position for a few minutes and then slowly rise.

Reiki Partner Meditation—Exercise III

This is a joint exercise for two people. Practise it with anyone who has become a channel for Reiki. It will help you experience your exercise partner on a level of reality that is beyond imagination. You learn to accept one another in a deep and loving manner and develop a greater understanding for each other stemming from this acceptance.

This is the ideal exercise for a loving couple, and will open new dimensions in the partnership. Practise it before sleeping with each other, or if you just want to lie together affectionately. It will arouse that deep trust in you without which sex and sensuality cannot really be enjoyed. It will allow total togetherness. Moreover, it also supplies all the bodily regions with Reiki via the reflex zones.

Sit facing each other on an even, not too pliable surface. Spread your legs a little wider apart than the width of your shoulders and draw up your knees. Now move close together so that one of you is able to put his or her legs over those of the other. Now join your palms (see Figure 39).

Your energy and Reiki energy now circulate between you and become enhanced in the process to an extent that amounts to more

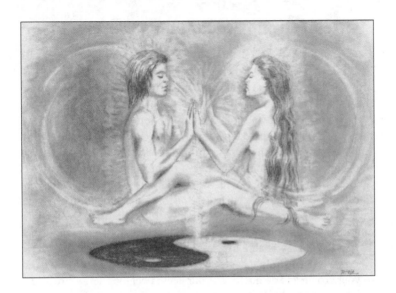

Fig. 39: Reiki partner meditation—exercise III

than just an addition of life forces. Feel your partner within you. Let Reiki energy flow through you, feel the resonance of the vibration in you and the warmth and presence of the loved one. If you prolong this meditation for any length of time, it will become a wonderful experience of emotional attachment beyond anything that can be experienced in day-to-day reality.

If you wish you may further extend your limits by intoning the mantra OM. Even if you start chanting separately, you will gradually come together through the rhythm of breathing, reflecting the merging of the two vibrations into a joint higher frequency. This process is, in the cosmic sense, the function of steady partnerships here on earth. By means of this simple exercise you can consciously experience your love and attachment and feel the support that the presence of the other gives you on this joint path to becoming One.

Five minutes are the absolute minimum for this exercise! Letting in, letting go, merging and finding your way back to yourself, infinitely enriched, takes some time. It cannot be done in a hurry, so 15 to 30 minutes are better. Reserve this time once or twice a week, just for yourselves; it will be worth it for both of you.

Reiki Group Meditation—Exercise IV

This is a group exercise that developed out of the well-known Energy Circle. There must be at least two participants, but a larger group makes it more beautiful.

Stand in a circle and join hands. The left hand (yin side of the body) is held with the palm turned upwards, the right hand (yang side of the body) with the palm turned downwards. The connection of energy circuits is most effective if palm is placed to palm.

Stand with your legs about as wide apart as your shoulders. Feel into your feet and feel your soles touching the ground. Keep your legs relaxed and bend the knees slightly (they should not be straight and stiff). Relax your pelvis and position it directly under your trunk so that the energy is able to rise unhindered from your root chakra. Keep your head straight as if it were drawn upward by a string fixed to your crown and do not touch your neck. Feel the energy streaming through your body; feel the flow and the vibration in yourself. Let yourself go and experience the sensations. Perceive the hands of the others to your right and left. Feel the Reiki energy flowing into them.

This group meditation may be extended by joint intoning of the mantra OM. I always find it a very special experience to be infused by the powerful vibration of OM in a Reiki energy circle with my body, becoming a sounding board for this powerful divine vibration of unconditional loving acceptance.

You may also make the exercise into a healing circle. After the energy circle has been upheld for some time, a member of the group leads everyone through the following visualization; imagine a white, divine light flowing into your crown chakra. It is flowing towards your heart, radiating from there as healing energy into the center of the circle. All the rays of energy meet there, forming a large, white mass of divine, healing vibrations. You may now place all those you wish to be healed into this energy mass simply by speaking their names. They will be given all the healing they need for the moment; all the healing which is advisable for them from a divine perspective. You may also place other beings into the circle (such as animals and plants). At the end take Mother Earth into the center of the healing circle and yourself. Now open yourself as much as you can to the energy of healing love. Let yourself be flooded by it and let every shadow you would like to let go of be transformed into radiant light. "Feel the energy ..."

The participants can remain infused by the healing force for as long as they wish. Eventually say farewell to the beings you called for healing, and bless them if you feel like it. At the end everybody reunites his astral body with the material body through visualization and slowly opens his eyes. The energy circle may now be slowly dissolved. If you wish you may give thanks for the beautiful experience, to others, to God, and to yourself before withdrawing your hands.

After some powerful group healing I like to lie down for a while, and feel into myself. Others joke or laugh or do other things that express their joy.

Summary
Reiki and Meditation

Exercise I: Enhancement of personal growth; developing the capacity of loving acceptance (correspondence with the rose quartz), practising a meditative mental attitude for day-to-day life; developing self-perception (especially in connection with the mantra OM; gradual, harmonious release of blockages; stress release; minimum duration three minutes, to be increased gradually.

Exercise II: Enhancement of personal growth; grounding; charging the root chakra; charging the aura; creating distance so as to be less sensitive (correspondence to lavender); minimum duration three minutes, to be increased gradually. This method is extremely suitable for healing the chakras.

Exercise III: Enhancement of a relationship on the emotional level; release of blockages in the region of the Third Eye and in the pelvic region; experience of oneness with a partner along with a simultaneous increase in vibrational frequency; strengthens the neck chakra. Pay attention to fears of physical closeness. If these are not released during the next exercise, help should be sought from a qualified therapist. (Don't try to force things!) Minimum duration five minutes, or better fifteen minutes.

Exercise IV: Enhancement of group consciousness; opening of the heart chakra; experience of oneness with other aspects of creation; increasing vibrational frequency; activating the body's self-healing forces. (Pay attention to fears of physical closeness. They occur only rarely in the energy circle, but nevertheless you should always be attentive when several people stand in close proximity for a longer period of time.) Minimum duration about five minutes, or preferably ten minutes.

Chapter Twelve

Reiki and Medication

Since Reiki is able to be given with great benefit as a supporting measure in the case of severe illnesses, it is important to know whether interactions with drugs may occur, and in what form.

There now follows a description of the experiences that therapists, Reiki lovers and practitioners of natural therapeutics have gathered in this area, including some observations of my own. The description is by no means complete, and it might be worth having some of them subjected to a series of tests. However, there is no need to wait for these tests to be carried out as the present state of knowledge already provides us with sufficient guidelines on how to use Reiki in conjunction with medication.

One essential effect of Reiki is that it supports all vital processes. It stimulates the metabolism and promotes detoxification. It induces a deep state of relaxation in the whole body, thus supporting the organism's responsiveness on all levels. Thus it is only logical that Reiki must have an effect on medication.

Chemical (Allopathic) Drugs

We are able to conclude from our experience that Reiki softens the effect of allopathic drugs that cause deliberate poisoning of the organism.(Reiki will reduce the side effects of such treatment, depending on the power and duration of Reiki treatment, and at a faster rate than is normally to be expected with these drugs). On the other hand it enhances receptivity, meaning if it is applied before the drug is taken, a lower dose will be sufficient for the desired effect. Naturally, this too depends on the duration and intensity of the previous Reiki session. This effect should also be taken into consideration with pain killers and anaesthetics which have to remain in the body at constant levels. There are certain local anaesthetics (as in dentistry) which contain special substances that constrict the blood vessels, thus keeping the anaesthetic substance in the narcotized area for a longer period of time. As Reiki causes a deep state of relaxation it will counteract the effect of the injection.

In Second Degree courses the Reiki teacher instructs participants never to use distance treatments on people undergoing operations, as the patient could wake up from anaesthesia prematurely. This also applies to First Degree treatment.

Anaesthesia and injections can be released from the system more harmoniously with Reiki once they have served their purpose. If powerful pain killers are given after the operation, you should avoid prolonged whole body treatment, giving Reiki only to the region of the body that has been operated on and to organs that are under special strain (for instance, the liver or the kidneys). I have observed, however, that the effect of a pain killer acting on the whole body is not reduced by Reiki. On the other hand, Reiki often stops or eases traumatic pain. You may also give Reiki to especially strained lymph nodes.

If there is minor pain, Reiki may often make anaesthetic medication superfluous. Headache and minor wounds, insect bites and sensitive teeth may be treated in this way without having to take recourse to pharmaceutical drugs.

Similar caution as with anaesthetic drugs is imperative for drugs that are only effective if maintained in certain quantities in the blood stream, such as anticoagulants and cardiac stimulants.

Be that as it may, I have heard some very positive reports on Reiki given before and after chemotherapy, but whole body treatment should be avoided during the actual course of chemotherapy. If in doubt, only apply Reiki whole body treatment in consultation with the specialist in charge, who obviously knows the effects of the prescribed drugs in detail. If he is open-minded, effective combinations of allopathic drugs and Reiki may be agreed.

Only very intensive Reiki whole body treatment has sufficient energy to reduce the effects of an allopathic drug considerably. However, since such treatment will also induce life-promoting processes, a drastic deterioration of the client's condition is hardly to be expected. These hints are primarily meant to clarify the potential effects of Reiki on allopathic medication. Please do not arrive at the conclusion that Reiki could cause serious or lasting disorders.

Phytotherapy (Herbal Medicine)

If officinal herbs are used holistically, that is to normalize the regulative systems of the organism, Reiki increases their effectiveness and accelerates the healing process. The application of synthetic or isolated herbal substances no longer containing the life force of a herb is equal to that of allopathic medication.

Homeopathy

Homeopathic remedies have a regulative effect on all dysfunctions of the organism on the physical and mental levels. If administered according to homeopathic principles, they are absolutely holistic in effect! Reiki enhances their action and can ease initial reactions and reduce their duration. In the case of treatment with detoxifying remedies such as Sulphur, Magnesium Fluoratum or nosodes, Reiki helps improve this process. On the other hand, specific Reiki work on the lymph node system and the eliminating organs can help prevent excessive strain and thus ensure gentle healing.

If low potencies (up to about D6, depending on the substance) are given in large doses, Reiki applications (especially whole body treat-

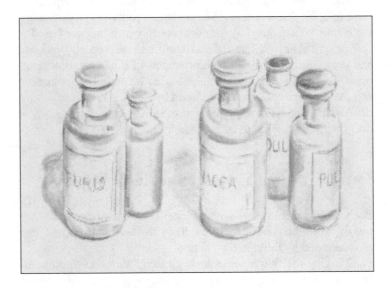

Fig. 40: Reiki and Medication

ment) stabilizes the physiological blood level of the respective substance(s) by accelerating the elimination of substances that are not wholesome for the body. If a substantial effect is intended, supporting Reiki treatment should take this into consideration accordingly.

Reiki often enhances the body's responsiveness in the case of homeopathic remedies, and frequent application, whether on the giving or receiving end, will make the organism more sensitive to their effects. With time, the prescriptions move in the direction of higher potencies and smaller doses and from animal substances to mineral and metallic ones. After prolonged Reiki application symptoms generally appear in a clearer form.

Homeopathy finds its limits wherever organisms cannot mobilize sufficient self-healing energy. Here Reiki whole body treatment and specific Reiki work on the root chakra may be of great help.

After prolonged homeopathic treatment, Reiki may also be applied along with the respective remedies to strengthen the organism, and thus shortens the convalescent period.

Spagyrism

This method of healing uses alchemic principles and techniques in the manufacture of drugs. The system used for the prescription of these remedies has a certain affinity to homeopathy and phytotherapy, but cannot be explained by the concepts on which they are based.

Spagyrism has a holistic effect if the drugs are properly produced and prescribed according to the principles of this method of treatment. According to accounts related to me, the period of application and the dose are considerably reduced by Reiki. As in homeopathy, detoxifying therapies are also supported, and charging spagyrical drugs with Reiki tends to increase their effect.

Flower Remedies

Bach, Californian, Australian and local flower remedies are effective on very high vibrational levels. They are absolutely holistic, and are supported by Reiki in their action.

Charging the flower remedies with Reiki increases them in effect, as does the use of special colored foils according to the Verana System®.(See the Appendix and List of Supply Sources).

One problem in applying the flower remedies is that the patient has to be attuned to high vibrations if the full action of the remedies is to unfold. Regular Reiki whole body treatment before and after taking the remedy may help the patient open to the high vibrational frequencies of the essences. Another possibility is specific Reiki work on the chakras addressed by the flowers.

Summary
Reiki and Medication

Allopathy: Never give Reiki in the case of anaesthesia; this is not permitted under any circumstances whatsoever. Also be careful in the case of pain killers and remedies that are required in the body at constant levels (such as anticoagulants and cardiac stimulants etc.). However, Reiki is able to prevent the damaging side effects of allopathic treatments.

Phytotherapy: Reiki has a supporting effect, but be careful in the case of isolated herbal ingredients. (The same restrictions apply as for allopathic drugs).

Homeopathy: Reiki has a supporting effect and enhances the body's responsiveness. Supports detoxifying therapies and is generally strengthening in effect, generally applied in high potencies at low doses with a shift towards mineral remedies.

Spagyrism: See Homeopathy; charging the drugs with Reiki increases their effect.

Flower remedies: See spagyrism; Reiki applied before and during administration improves the body's responsiveness; Vera colored foils increase the power of the remedies.

Chapter Thirteen

Reiki with Plants and Animals

Naturally, Reiki energy is not just available to humans. Animals and plants can also benefit by it and enjoy receiving it and feeling its flow. Of course Reiki work with animals is slightly different from that with human clients. Here are some hints.

Reiki and Plants

Since plants come in a variety of sizes, that is from a few millimeters (seeds) to several hundred feet (sequoias), different periods of time are required for their treatment. A period of about two to three minutes for seeds and five to ten minutes for room plants has been found to be effective. Larger plants can generally not be helped by First Degree treatment. Second Degree Reiki is more appropriate, as is also the case with whole forests, which can be supplied with Reiki energy in this manner both quickly and easily. If we wish to supply large plants or a small garden with Reiki, the easiest way is to charge the water. In my experience one or two minutes per quart are sufficient. Whether the charge is sufficient or not can easily be tested with a pendulum; if the pendulum provides no more evidence of negative vibrations, the water can be used.

You should always treat the roots of house plants, not only the leaves. If transmitted to the roots, Reiki is a remedy against soft rot, whether for its prevention or healing. Regular applications of Reiki to the root system encourage freshly repotted plants to spread their roots in the new soil and adapt to their new environment.

Reiki and Pests

If plants are infested by pests, you can effectively help them with Reiki. A few minutes of treatment will mostly be sufficient to increase the vitality of house plants so that they are able to form enough resistance to parasites. As a rule, the pests will have already dropped

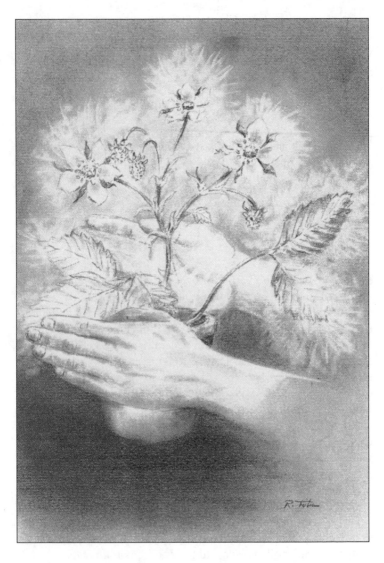

Fig. 41: Reiki for house plants

off the next day. However, since parasites pass on poisonous substances into the earth, thereby continuing to affect the plant even after their removal, we should wash the leaves thoroughly. Apply some more Reiki over the next few days more to revitalize the plant. This is very important as it may otherwise not stand the strain of the defensive reaction, especially in the case of abundant infestation.

Reiki Meditation with Trees

Trees act as wonderful companions for meditation. Stand close to a strong tree and place your palms on its trunk or embrace it. After a while you will sense its powerful, calm presence. During this process you give it Reiki and the tree takes you into its aura. If you do this regularly with a particular tree, it may reveal images or other impressions. Trees can be good advisers if they trust you. If you now think I've gone slightly mad, just try it—you will be as surprised as I was when I first made contact with a tree.

Reiki and Acid Rain

In this day and age it is very important to remember that we humans should not use the world like a self-service shop along the lines of "just throw it away, tomorrow the shelves will be refilled". This attitude has already caused immeasurable damage. If you have been initiated into Second Degree Reiki, you can do a lot to help trees live (and survive). Find out which particular forests near your home are especially damaged and send them regular Reiki energy via distance treatment. It will be even better if you are joined by friends who can also administer Second Degree Reiki. This kind of "tree support group" is often able to accomplish small miracles. If you are interested in environmental work with Reiki, I would be happy if you would send me a note. I will collect the addresses and pass them on to interested people (only if you grant your consent, of course). If you have had some experience with this kind of Reiki application, I would appreciate it if you would share it with me. Perhaps I could take it into consideration in future editions of the book. Indeed, maybe a Reiki environmental network would evolve with time. It would be of good use to the world.

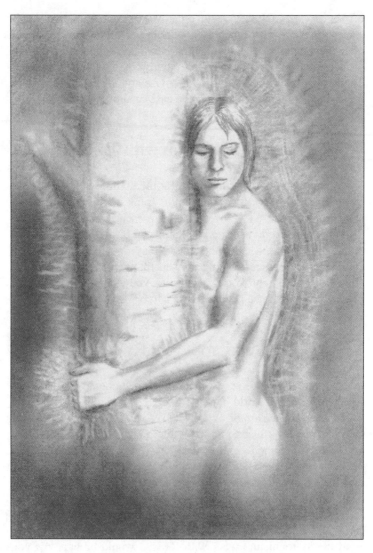

Fig. 42: Reiki exchange with a tree

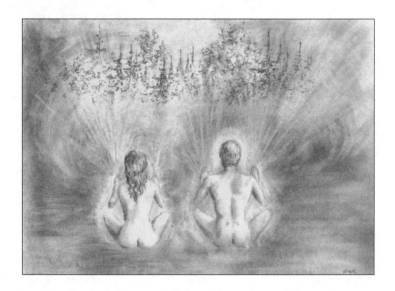

Fig. 43: Distance Reiki to support the dying forests

Reiki and Animals

All animals like Reiki. They are very sensitive to the energy and know exactly how much and at which part of the body they need it, In other words, it is they that determine the duration and the priorities of Reiki sessions.

This is how a Reiki session with an animal can typically take place; you are having a cup of tea with a friend. Suddenly your dog comes up to you, prods you with its nose and leans against you. If you now place your hands on the dog, it will position itself in such a way that they touch the right spot. Once it gets restless or goes away, the session is over.

Such Reiki sessions will affect your relationship to the animal concerned. I have seen true friendships developing as a result of these Reiki treatments. The animals lose their natural shyness and become very trusting.

Large or dangerous animals should only be provided with Second Degree distant treatment. If that is not possible, you can at least charge their food and drinking water with Reiki before they are fed. The effect is less than that of direct Reiki treatment, but if done regularly over a long period of time, this will also be of help. As for the feed, our domestic animals are normally given factory-produced food and tap water. Both are not exactly ideal for their well-being. If it is not possible to provide healthier food (such as fresh meat and or spring water), you can at least charge the food with Reiki. This reduces the effect of harmful substances and the food is more easily digested. Incidentally, the same is also true for your own food.

Reiki and Horses

I have learned from a friend who is a veterinary practitioner of natural therapeutics that she is cures horses of troublesome colic a lot faster with Reiki. If Reiki energy is given along with homeopathic remedies, there is often an improvement within quarter of an hour. She simply places her hands on the horse's stomach and after a while changes to another area.

Reiki and Cats

Castration is almost inevitable for domestic tomcats. Cats are often sterilized so that they aren't constantly on heat and suffer accordingly. With the help of Reiki you are able to help your feline companions to cope with the operation and shorten the period of convalescence. Cats on heat become more peaceful if they receive a lot of Reiki during this time. It also helps if you chant the vowel "ooo" from the depths of your stomach. The vibration of this vowel corresponds to the sexual center and gets the animal in touch with the energy it desires. But it only works if the sound is really formed in your stomach; if it isn't, the vibration of the second chakra will be missing. If your friends think you are crazy when you intone a deep abdominal "ooo", don't worry. They'll get used to it. Perhaps they'll even adopt the method after seeing that it works.

Basically, Reiki has its effect on all beings in your environment. Plants and animals will feel good in your presence and encounter you with greater trust. Your hand chakras are constantly passing Reiki into your aura, and therefore whatever comes into contact with your aura also comes into contact with Reiki. You may notice that your hands start to tingle when you are near certain plants or animals. This means that they are absorbing a dose of life energy from you.

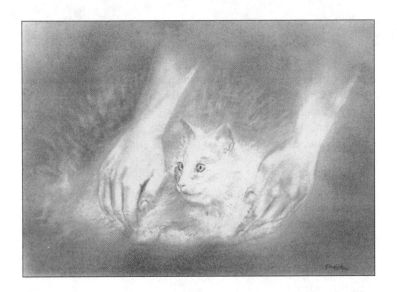

Fig. 44: Cats like Reiki

It may well be that your pet will be a little confused by your Reiki attunement. It can feel the change in your vibrations and is unable to understand it at first. It will soon come up to you and will soon be snuggling your hands.

Summary
Reiki with Plants and Animals

Plants can be provided with direct treatment of their leaves and roots or the water you give them. Second Degree Reiki can be used to supply a number of plants with Reiki energy at the same time. Treat small, young or weak plants for only short periods at first and then gradually increase. Use distance treatment for forests weakened by acid rain.

Animals may be treated directly, unless they are dangerous. Provide large and dangerous animals with distance treatment or simply treat their food and water. Animals generally determine for themselves how long they want Reiki, and where. Pay attention to this and re-spect their decision. Animals often react in a confused way when a familiar person has been initiated into Reiki, but will soon return of their own accord.

Chapter Fourteen

The Possibilities of Second and Third Degree Reiki

Second Degree Reiki implies an amplification of your capacities on all levels. Certain things you only read in fantasy novels or see in the movies become true through the possibilities of the Second Degree.

In this chapter I will be relating some of the things that Second and Third Degree Reiki make possible. I will not be able to go into specific detail, however, as information on practical application is only transferred orally and I do not wish to break with this tradition.

Second Degree Reiki is accompanied by a great deal of power. Only a person who works with a trained Reiki master should have access to the symbols and techniques that are a part of it.

The flow of Reiki energy can be increased many times with the help of these techniques, making it easier to cleanse objects on an energetic level. The sessions become shorter in length, and their effect greater.

Another Second Degree technique facilitates harmonization on the mental and emotional level, meaning that Reiki is able to reach the subconscious directly. Karmic patterns, fears, addiction and other mental disorders will be affected positively. You can also provide objects, especially precious stones and certain metals, with positive energy. Processes of growing awareness are also accelerated.

The last basic Second Degree technique, now to be described, may also be the one with the most varied possibilities, in that it can be used to send Reiki to any place across distance and any time. Since the connection works both ways, with a little practise you can also exchange information this way. You can clean the energy in rooms, neutralize earth and other radiation (to a certain degree) and set up Reiki "showers" at certain places. Whole countries, even the whole earth, can be supplied with Reiki. Quantities of energy will be small, of course, but if a large group of people with Second Degree initiation collaborate, anything is possible. In the fall of 1989, a world-wide action of this kind was staged for political reasons.

These abilities may be used for the good of others but also for improving your own health and development. For example, you are able to supply your whole body with Reiki on the basis of distance

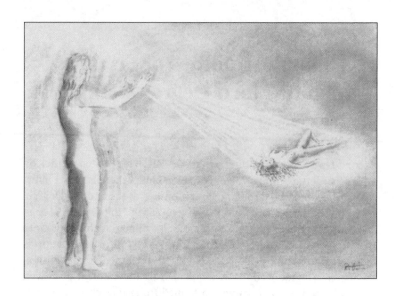

Fig. 45: Reiki distance treatment

treatment. The period required is only about 20 minutes. As a comparison, First Degree contact treatment takes about 90 minutes. You can also transmit Reiki to several people at the same time with Second Degree Reiki.

Another possibility is to transmit Reiki into particular formative situations of the past, thus dissolving patterns and opening up new avenues of development.

So much on this subject. If you would like to know more, contact a Reiki master. And if you believe that all this is less than plausible, ask someone who has received Second Degree initiation to do distance energy transmission on you. Then you will know for yourself.

Third Degree Reiki

This is the Master Degree, and those who are initiated into it are able to help others become a Reiki channel, although not themselves. Even Reiki masters are "just" channels of Universal Life Energy. Many personal processes of transformation are connected with the Master Degree, and therefore initiation requires a very close inner connection with Reiki. Hawaya Takata, the Grand Master before last, once expressed it this way; "If you are ready to give up everything to take Reiki into the world, you are ready to become a Reiki Master!" Reiki masters are not committed to any particular group, are absolutely free in their decisions and their religious faith. Neither are they under the control of the respective Grand Master.

In other words, Reiki is neither a sect nor a church, and there is no Reiki guru to call the tune and point the way. The message of Reiki energy is love and freedom, not dependence and dogma.

Chapter Fifteen

Questions and Answers

"How is it that I sometimes don't feel anything in my hands?"

There could be several reasons. If you are involved in hectic day-to-day living, you generally become less sensitive in order to cope with all the impressions flooding in on you from your surroundings without becoming overly distracted. This, however, lowers your sensitivity to the more subtle sensations (such as the flow of Reiki energy.) In other words, you will hardly notice the flow of Reiki, or not notice it at all. If you give yourself some time to relax, you will begin to get a feeling for the energy again.

Another reason may be that you are fairly new to First Degree Reiki. Your perceptive faculties may not have had a chance to develop sufficiently to perceive Reiki, but if you work with it regularly, this will change. Just take your time and practice the sensitizing techniques described in Chapter Seven.

Finally, the reason might be that the energy isn't flowing at all. As you know, Reiki is drawn or "sucked in" by the recipient. If he has some unconscious block or simply does not require any energy, there may be no flow, which is perhaps why you do not sense anything. If there is a local blockage, you can treat this area of the body via the reflex zones. The further away the zones are from the blocked area, the better.

"Will the channel ever close or Reiki stop flowing?"

No, this is not possible. Through the four initiations you become a Reiki channel and stay connected with this divine energy for the rest of your life. Even if you don't use Reiki for 20 years (which actually is impossible as Reiki flows automatically the moment you place your hands on something requiring Reiki), it is as freely available as after your initiation. It may well be that you simply are not able to perceive the energy at the moment for some reason (see above).

"How is it that sometimes nothing seems to happen when I give Reiki?"

Something always happens when Reiki flows into a living being, but perhaps something quite different to what you expected. Reiki always acts in its own way and you can only influence this within narrow boundaries. The following example illustrates this point; perhaps you want to help someone stop smoking, and although you give him Reiki, nothing happens. However, your client suddenly starts to enjoy exercise and play tennis a few weeks later. Perhaps this was more important, and perhaps stopping smoking was not as urgent as both of you thought.

If you treat an acute physical disorder with Reiki and there are no evident results, a trained medical specialist should be consulted without delay. It is possible that there is not enough Reiki to change things for the better, or that there is some organic disorder requiring surgical or other treatment. When pus is involved or severe, constant pain, the client should be referred to a physician or a practitioner of natural therapeutics without any further experimentation. Reiki does not make emergency measures superfluous.

"Does Reiki amount to faith healing?"

There is no simple answer to this question. There are so many methods of faith healing, from the "faith surgeons" in Brazil to healing with "the Energy of Christ" and so on. All of these can be called faith healing as they work with subtle energies that somehow address the whole person in the healing process. This is also what Reiki does, but basically its use as a means of healing physical disorders is only a small facet of its many possibilities. Every person is able to use Reiki to live more consciously, become more perceptive and alive or simply to sense God's presence. Reiki is not simply—as other methods of faith healing—a way of bringing health to the ill but also and to a much greater extent a means for people without complaints to develop their vitality and capacity to love in a simple and lasting manner (see Chapter One).

Perhaps the question can be answered in this way; faith healing is just one of the many possibilities of Reiki.

"My wife/daughter/mother/aunt would so much benefit from Reiki, but whenever I ask her she does not want to be treated or be initiated. Should I let myself be initiated into the Second Degree so that I can treat her via distance healing? She couldn't do anything about that, could she?

Reiki should not be forced onto any living being against its declared will. After all, every person is entitled to his or her own way of life. Second Degree Reiki is not meant to be used contrary to the wishes or intentions of another. By declared will I don't mean that the person concerned owes you an explanation, rather what I am referring to is any clear expression of refusal, even in the form of an unmistakable gesture (as with animals).

This point is especially important for those initiated into Second Degree Reiki because they are able to transmit Reiki energy anywhere they like without having direct contact with the recipient. If you are not able to determine whether the potential recipient is in agreement with treatment (due to coma, unconsciousness, mental imbalance, no possibility of contact or similar), you should consult an oracle or decide on a distance treatment according to your intuition and in a responsible manner.

"Why are the Reiki initiations so expensive?"

1. Every person just needs one initiation for each Reiki Degree for his whole life, so relatively speaking, the expense is minimal. If you consider the cost-benefit ratio, you will probably come to the conclusion that the initiations should actually be more expensive.
2. Since each person is only initiated into each Reiki Degree once, and since Reiki masters also have to make their living and recover costs, obviously Reiki cannot be had at a bargain price.
3. A Reiki initiation is a wonderful thing, but people are able to also live quite happily without it. In other words, people are not withheld something that they absolutely need by the price. If you need Reiki for your personal development, you will be able to afford it.
4. The course fees are ultimately regulated by the market, as are all other prices for goods and services. There is no such thing as a "just price". A price is justified whenever a sufficient number of customers accept it, and a sufficient number of suppliers deliver.
5. Reiki represents a certain value, and people tend to take a more respectful attitude to things that cost a lot of money. Since Reiki becomes as much a part of a person as his inborn talents, it is important to regard Reiki as valuable from the onset. After all, we are very

reluctant to accept the parts of our personality that we see as being of no great value. Only in extremely rare cases do I give a discount on my Reiki course fees. Hawayo Takata, the Grand Master before last, gave the subject short shrift—"Don't bargain with Reiki!". That's exactly the way I feel about it too. There's something not quite right about bargaining with Reiki.

"Is it absolutely necessary to have a Reiki initiation to be able to lay on hands?"

No, of course not. Basically, every human has the capacity to transmit life energy through his hands, some a little more than others. However, Reiki initiations guarantee that it is not your life energy that is being transmitted, but Universal Life Energy. It is rather that Universal Life Energy is being channelled. It is because of this that Reiki does not cause fatigue and that no specific exercises are need to be performed to gain the energy in the first place. Moveover, Reiki initiation helps set up mechanisms that protect you and the client from negative vibrations. Furthermore, each initiation multiplies the capacity for transmitting energy many times. Traditional Reiki initiation is accompanied by further effects, but these are discussed elsewhere in this book.

"Do I need to have faith in Reiki to make it work?"

No, Reiki is automatically transmitted if it is needed and is accepted by the subconscious. Reiki is not a psychological phenomenon like hypnosis or suggestion. The effects of Reiki cannot be explained by the placebo effect or other suggestive effects. The energy flows, even if the Reiki channel does not believe in anything in particular. It all takes place automatically without any prerequisites.

"Is Reiki magic?"

A definition of magic that I find pretty appropriate has been put as follows, although the quote may not be 100 % correct; "Magic is the art of bringing about changes of consciousness at will" (Dion Fortune). According to this definition Reiki cannot be magic, because processes that result in a higher degree of awareness proceed on their own, according to their own dynamic laws and therefore cannot be influenced by will. It is the flow of life energy which sets them in motion.

Common parlance defines magic as "the art of using natural forces and means to achieve amazing results." According to this definition, Reiki is indeed magic. If the question "Is Reiki magic?" has anything to do with black magic, let me reassure you that this is not the case.

The essence of Reiki is unlimited love. So-called black magic is ultimately based on the power of hatred and fear.

"What actually happens at the initiations that take place at Reiki seminars?"

At the initiations the Reiki Master acts as a channel and mediator of Universal Life Energy. If you think this sounds a bit far-fetched, all I can say is that there is no other way of putting it. This contact with the divine force is so profound that it reaches you in your innermost core. It is at this level that you are freed of ideas of guilt—a necessary step in becoming a channel of Universal Life Energy. This is why the traditional initiation steps bring about such an increase in one's capacity for love and consciousness. The ritual performed as part of each initiation is like a key agreed on with God for unlocking the power of healing love.

"Can I harm anyone with Reiki?"

No, you can't. Reiki is love, and love does not harm anyone. But if you fall prey of the delusion of power of being able to heal everything and everyone with "your" Reiki energy, and do not fetch or carry out the necessary medical or therapeutic help in situations requiring it, your wish to exercise power will indeed cause harm. Reiki does not relieve you of the responsibility toward yourself and those who entrust themselves to you.

"Does Reiki only flow if I first pray and then smooth out the aura?"

Reiki always flows wherever it is needed and wherever it is accepted. There are no any other preconditions. Reiki is a gift. There are no strings attached.

"Is it possible to cure every type of health disorder with Reiki?"

No it isn't. Reiki can do a lot but it can't do everything and it does not make conventional or naturopathic therapies and diagnosis superfluous either, but simply provides them with appropriate support. Symptoms of serious disease or anything similar should be treated by trained medical specialists. In the hands of laymen, Reiki should mainly be used as a prophylactic measure or as a means of treating trivial complaints (which one usually treats oneself without consulting a physician practitioner of natural therapeutics). However, Reiki can be of great help as a supporting measure for treatment of all kinds.

"Whenever I give myself Reiki, it doesn't work. Why not?"

Reiki does not impair your individual freedom of choice. If you consciously or subconsciously want someone else to take care of you, you will close yourself off to your "own" Reiki. In this case you are not interested in having the problem solved, but in satisfying your desire for closeness. This is perfectly legitimate and you should accept it if it is indeed the case. Reiki cannot and should not replace human closeness.

"Does the same quantity of Reiki flow in everyone?"

No, it does not. The initiations greatly enhance the capacity of each person to pass on life energy and lifts them to a level where certain effects become possible. This is the basic opening up that takes place, and it can never be reduced. If you give a lot of Reiki, your capacity to channel this energy will also be increased. This too will become part of you and cannot be withdrawn or limited.

Through the initiations into the Second and Third Degree, the opening for the Universal Life Energy is developed further each time. The flow of energy can be further enhanced with the Second Degree symbols.

"Recently, I have been feeling tired whenever I give a lot of Reiki. What's the cause?"

Whenever you pass on Reiki to another, you also get your own share of the energy. Cleansing processes are instigated in your own body the moment you lay your hands on another person. The healing reaction then consumes the body's energies while it is acting. Give yourself plenty of Reiki to help your organism and give yourself time and leisure to grow. The more you work with Reiki, the less "energy-sapping" reactions will occur. Your energy channels will become more and more open and efficient (also see the question above).

"Can the Reiki initiation be reversed?"

No, it can't. The Reiki initiations are carried out by God, and the Reiki Masters themselves are just a channel through which this power is able to pass. Man and God stand in constant contact during the initiation. External factors and phenomena of whatever kind cannot influence God. Reiki initiations cannot be made ineffective through some presumed guilt or lapse or other "moral" reasons, either.

"I feel Reiki does me a lot of good, but I simply don't take the time to treat myself. Why am I like this?"

What kind of relationship do you have to yourself? Is it loving? Do you allow yourself some of the good things in life? This is often not the case in this kind of situation. What might be helpful are affirmations such as "I allow time for myself because I love myself!" or "I love myself and enjoy doing myself some good". Working with rose quartz is also helpful. Take some time and sit down and begin to think about why you don't take the time to treat yourself. Look for the real reasons, and ignore the famous excuse "I simply don't have the time". This is often the first step to solving the problem. If that doesn't help, then give into your feelings and take care of others until you're utterly fed up with it and just want time to yourself. I have found that this has always done the trick. Anyone with the "Good Samaritan syndrome" will have to face up to this question sooner or later, or just burn up.

There's also another possibility. You might simply be overwhelmed by the speed of your own growth, or by the possibilities that open up to you. Since Reiki is something that stimulates growth, you are trying to avoid it. Take a rest for a while. If you like, look into your fear of development. Your desire to give Reiki will return with time. Both rest and exercise have their purpose, one cannot exist without the other.

"I'm afraid of interfering with my karma or that of other people with Reiki. Is this possible?"

The essence of Reiki is love and you cannot do anything wrong with that. If some karmic burden is to be released through Reiki, that's great stuff. It is impossible to create new burdens of this kind with Reiki, unless the person applying it wants to live out his need for power. One should make a clear distinction between the two. If I try to treat someone against his will I am creating karma, but not for the other person, only for myself. The power of Reiki makes sure of this.

"Why do I need all these methods with precious stones and scents and meditation? Doesn't Reiki work just as well on its own?"

Of course it does, but in order to achieve anything it first has to be applied and then it has to be accepted and let in. Since some people prefer to be treated with Reiki when it is packaged in a nice way and since our subconscious often wants to be made a fuss of and stimulated before it is ready to let in Reiki, the methods described in this book can make a considerable indirect contribution to the effectiveness of Reiki. I am not a purist and therefore I choose my methods according to effectiveness. This does not necessarily have to apply to you, however. Do whatever you like as long as you enjoy doing it and it doesn't deprive others of their possibilities or development.

Chapter Sixteen

My Personal Contact and Growth with Reiki

You have probably now read the "Reiki Handbook" or at least leafed through it and browsed through one section or another. Perhaps you would like to know how I got to know Reiki and what working with it means to me personally. Such accounts are also helpful and that is my intention.

Like many others, I became acquainted with Reiki and naturopathy because of personal problems and because conventional medicine was not able to offer any solutions.

A few years ago I was in extremely bad health. On waking up every morning I felt exhausted and I only got through the day by drinking lots of coffee. In the evenings I didn't feel like doing anything.

I consulted three physicians, one after the other. They all told me the same thing, and that there was nothing wrong with me, at least nothing they could find, and apart from which, what could you expect at the age of 25—that's when the first signs of wear and tear appear. At first I thought they were joking. But no, they meant it seriously.

After following various other wrong tracks, I finally came across the practice of Horst Kosche, a naturopath. It was there for the first time that I got to know applied naturopathics. By means of careful iris diagnosis and blood test, he found that some metabolic disease was the cause of my problems and he then began an appropriate course of treatment with great success.

During the treatment I often had the opportunity to talk with him and his wife Sabine. With time I came to see myself and my health from another, more holistic perspective.

One day I discovered a First Degree Reiki certificate in the waiting room. I was already familiar with acupuncture, chiropractic and homeopathy, but Reiki? I had no idea. I had never heard the word before.

I asked about it and was told that there would soon be another Reiki seminar in one of the consulting rooms, and that it would be worth my while to take part.

Without knowing much about Reiki, I enrolled. Then one spring Friday evening I went to the seminar with Manu, who was my girl-friend at the time and who is now my wife.

About 20 people were already there, some of whom seemed very exotic. But the most exotic of all appeared to be Brigitte Müller, the Reiki master conducting the seminar. Dressed in various shades pur-ple (and very elegant as well), she did not quite tally with the idea I had at the time of a seminar leader.

I found the seminar very interesting because many new things were discussed. A dowser, for example, talked about his experiences during the breaks and introduced us to the possibilities of dowsing. Others told us about a Huna seminar they had recently attended, and a very fashionable young woman talked about her experiences as a faith healer.

These people also had some very strange ways of relating to one another. They all hugged as a welcome, even the men! The atmos-phere was warm and loving and the people dealt with each other in a relaxed and amicable way.

I did not experience anything extraordinary through the initia-tion. I felt a something tweaking or buzzing inside me whenever Brigitte placed her hands on me during the initiation ritual, but I didn't see any lights or hear any voices.

I was a bit disappointed. I would liked to have had some divine revelation, preferably in 3-D, with the Berlin Philharmonic orches-tra playing in the background. Nothing of the sort happened. Nor did I feel any tingling in my hands. The others talked about what they had experienced and had it interpreted by Brigitte, but I didn't feel anything.

Feeling confused and a bit disappointed (For heaven's sake, why wasn't there any tingling in my hands!), I left the seminar room on the Sunday afternoon with my certificate and the Reiki documents. "Well, it was great, especially because of all those crazy people!" I thought, "But otherwise it was a rather expensive weekend."

Next morning, when driving to work in my car, I began to feel very strange. As soon as I touched anything for more than a few seconds, my hands start to tingle and I felt a strange pulling and flowing feeling I had never felt before. If I kept my hands on any-thing for any length of time, my arms began to tingle right up to my shoulders as if they had pins and needles, but there was not the slight-est feeling of numbness you usually have with pins and needles.

Something had happened during the weekend after all!

I had a similar surprise later in the therapy group I had been at-tending for some time. Before the seminar I had found it difficult to have a casual relationship with the others in the group or to show any affection, but now suddenly I was able to take a woman who was crying into my arms and console her. Beforehand I would have spent so much time thinking about whether it was all right to comfort her or not or whether I ought to do so, that in the end she wouldn't have been crying any more. Suddenly I found it much easier to show my feelings.

During the next few months I gave Reiki a lot. Manu and I often gave each other a lot of Reiki too to share our new ability. It was such a beautiful experience to give and receive Reiki.

In spite of my constant dealings with the energy and its effects, I had to keep telling myself that it was really Reiki that was making all this happen whenever I laid my hands somewhere. I kept my hands on my body whenever possible in order to feel the energy and often treated the plants in our apartment whenever I felt the Reiki particularly clearly.

My doubts were finally dissolved by a somewhat dramatic event.

One day Manu had severe pain in the lower part of her abdomen. She was hardly able to walk and every twinge of pain made her jump. A visit to her physician and examination of the pelvic region produced the diagnosis of serious inflammation in the region of the left ovary. Manu had spent several weeks in hospital the previous year because of a similar complaint and was now very much afraid of an operation and antibiotic treatment. Moreover, we had planned to go on vacation a few days later. This would have had to have been cancelled if she didn't get better in time. The diagnosis was made on a Monday afternoon and Manu was told to see her gynaecologist the next day to be admitted into hospital.

We had already tried Reiki, of course, but it had brought about no results worth mentioning. So, faced with this acute problem, we remembered our Reiki master Brigitte Müller. When she introduced us to First Degree Reiki she mentioned that people initiated into the Second Degree could transmit Reiki over any distance without having physical contact, and increase it enormously by means of another technique. Since we didn't know anyone else who had the Second Degree, we called her and asked her for distance treatment the same evening. Manu laid down at the agreed time, and at the same time I gave her Reiki on her stomach. Nothing much happened for the first five minutes, but when suddenly the energy surged up my arms like a wave and passed to my heart region. Manu felt great warmth and a strong flow of energy in her stomach. We had never experienced that much Reiki energy before. After three quarters of an hour we finished the session and went to sleep.

When I went to work the next morning, Manu was still asleep as she did not have to go to the gynaecologist until later, but when we talked on the phone at noon, she was totally excited. Her gynaecologist had found that her clinical readings had returned to normal!

The X ray and the other examinations were also negative and best of all, Manu hadn't had any more pain at all since waking. She could walk again and climb stairs without difficulty. Obviously, the inflammation had healed entirely overnight.

We had a wonderful and peaceful vacation in France and from then on we knew that we would be taking part in the next seminar for Second Degree Reiki initiation together. From then on, Reiki would be a permanent part of our life.

Much has happened since then. We did the Second Degree together and have often had occasion to wonder at the effect of Reiki on both ourselves and others. Many of our little complaints have disappeared and our health has improved more and more. Healing with our hands soon became such an everyday occurrence that we stopped wondering whether Reiki would work this time or not. By now we were preoccupied with other and deeper processes of growth.

I began to feel a great desire to become a Reiki master myself, and I wanted to help pass on this wonderful ability that had helped me and others so much. Over the course of a year I was then trained by Brigitte Müller, whom the Reiki Grand Master Phyllis Furumoto had provided with permission to instruct and initiate masters.

This master training was quite different from what I expected. My image of a Reiki master was an inflexible and rigid one. During training I gained a better understanding of the responsibilities and possibilities of a Reiki master, during the course of which I became aware that there is no such thing as the "ideal Reiki Master". I had to explore my own inner potential and Brigitte was of great help here. She didn't shy away from confrontation and made no concessions in demonstrating her path as a Reiki Master.

She was a good example in that I learned not to have an example. Her style of teaching Reiki is not mine. She isn't any better or worse, but simply different. The way she does things is her way, that's all. This process of self-realization helped me to let go of my projections and find myself.

In this way I also arrived at new conclusions about the effects of initiation, namely that a process of healing and growth occurs with every Reiki initiation. Of course, everyone carries his own burdens and latent illnesses within himself, all aspects in requirement of healing. This means he will grow in a different way to other people.

Not everyone who has been initiated into the Second Degree is automatically healthier or wiser than someone who "only" has the First Degree.

Reiki masters too aren't necessarily further on the path than someone without Reiki or First or Second Degree. There are so many ways of learning and growing. It is just one of them, a very effective, safe and very beautiful one, but it is only one of the many developed by man with God's help.

I try to convey this view of things in my seminars, because it is so important for people to accept themselves the way they are and not make their self-esteem dependent on degrees or diplomas.

Reiki can contribute to every method of healing and growth. It can act as a turbocharger and accelerate processes of self-discovery. However, like all techniques of enhancing growth and self-discovery, it does not replace life itself. It increases your vitality and understanding of life, but it is not a substitute for experience or contact with others. A wise man once said that enlightenment cannot be achieved by eating the correct diet, by doing the right things, by practising meditation or any other deliberate means. We are here on earth to experience life, not to just meditate, share Reiki and think of nothing else but entering nirvana.

Enlightenment is a gift. It comes to us if we have experienced life fully and intensely. It comes naturally when it is the right time in the holistic sense.

If you accept Reiki as an assistant its energy will always be there to help you in your responsibilities. If you cannot accept Reiki as a path, there are many others and I hope you find the right one reliably and quickly. Never allow anyone convince you that you are worth less because you have not had this or that particular training.

This book brings a long-cherished wish to fruition. Ever since I became a Reiki channel, I had so many questions, but generally there was nobody there who could answer them. So I had to look for the answers myself. The topics discussed in this book are the result of many talks, books, seminars and simply experience. When I talked to other people about my experiences with Reiki, I noticed that they became more enthusiastic about working with it. They were able to use it in a more meaningful manner and by getting to know the Reiki philosophy were able to judge its possibilities and limitations more realistically. This inspired me to start teaching Reiki-Do, the path of healing love, and to provide guidance on practical Reiki work to interested friends in seminar form.

After I became a Reiki master, I immediately began to develop an advanced course for other people seeking this knowledge, and it is this which led on to this book. I hope it has clarified a lot of the questions that cannot be dealt with in Reiki seminars due to the lack of time, and I will be glad to receive any reader's letters to help me improve the manual. In case of interest, I can also imagine that some sections might be appended in future. So get your pens ready.

By the way, I have deliberately avoided using he/she and so on, as I think this only makes things more clumsy. I am a man and therefore I use the male case when I write. A woman would probably do the same by using the female case. That's all.

Wishing you love and light on your path

Walter Lübeck

Appendix

Therapeutic Index

This index is a list of symptoms and the positions suitable for treating them. Some whole treatment positions have proved to be particularly effective for certain symptoms, and can be maintained during whole body treatment for a longer period or applied separately.

A general rule is that complaints require a small number of sessions, but at frequent intervals. Chronic diseases should be treated at first with at least four successive whole body treatments, and then one to three times a week depending on the seriousness of the illness. You can calculate about one month of regular Reiki sessions per year that the illness has persisted (or a little more or less depending on the person's constitution and the state of the illness). Keep in mind that often decades pass before a cancerous disease really breaks out. The latent phase can be very long and we have to consider this when determining the period of treatment. Generally speaking the organism will not be capable of undergoing radical changes within a mere matter of weeks. In order to enable it to do this in the first place, the personality of the client has to change first and then slowly grow out of the illness. This takes time and regular treatment.

In the case of life-threatening diseases, chakra balancing and specific Reiki work on the first and sixth chakras is also important.

In the case of all diseases that disfigure in any way, chakra balancing and specific Reiki work on the second and fifth chakras should also be included.

Chakra balancing and specific work on the first, third and fifth chakras should be performed for all diseases which impair or paralyse the body or mind entirely or partially.

For all diseases of body liquids (blood/lymph/saliva/digestive juices/perspiration/dry skin/urine/diarrhoea/constipation), specific Reiki work on the kidneys and the second chakra should be included in treatment. For all nervous and mental diseases, include specific treatment of the solar plexus, hara and liver region.

Reiki treatment is no substitute for consultation of a physician, a practitioner of natural therapeutics or a psychotherapist! Serious diseases and any condition that could develop into a serious disease should be diagnosed and treated by competent specialists!

Accidents: Call a physician! As a first aid treat the shock with positions 13 and 8. Keep hands at a little distance directly over areas of potential internal bleeding, but in no case touch these areas (also see Panic and Fear.

Acne: Begin with whole body treatment on consecutive days. Then channel Reiki locally, daily or at least every second day, to the focus of the condition and use positions 5, 6, 8, 10 and 13.

Acute temper: Channel Reiki in at the wrists, on the top of the feet and a handsbreadth above the ankles and apply position 8. Treat tendency to temper with positions 6, 8, 11 and 14.

Addiction: The German word for addiction (Sucht) is derived from "suchen" (to search). Therefore do specific Reiki work on the sixth chakra (Third Eye). Apply whole body treatment for physical and mental detoxification. Also use positions 1, 5, 6, 8, 11, 12 and 13.

AIDS: Daily whole body treatment is absolutely necessary! Additionally employ positions 8, 9, 10, 13, 14 and 17.

Allergies: Begin therapy with whole body treatment. Then channel Reiki locally to the focus of the disease and use positions 1, 5, 8 and 10.

Amputations: Treat the stump and the artificial limb (as if it were the severed limb) and use positions 1, 8 and 14.

Anaemia: Give a few whole body treatments; after this apply positions 4, 6 and 7 and channel Reiki at the top of the head.

Anaesthesia: Never apply Reiki during anaesthesia under any circumstances whatsoever, as it could stop working. Whole body treatment before and after, and positions 1, 6, 8, 14 and 17. You can also (depending on the condition of your client) work with these positions alone and not carry out whole body treatment.

Angina Pectoris: Channel in Reiki at the diaphragm and upper back and apply positions 2, 3, 5 and 8.

Antibiotics (side effects): Give whole body treatment on consecutive days and positions 5, 6, 8, 9, 10 and 13 afterwards. Once the acute condition has cleared up, treat the liver and kidneys separately for some time once or twice a week and also employ position 17.

Appendicitis (also see Inflammation): Call a physician immediately and treat locally until he arrives; in the case of extreme pain apply positions and 17 (halfway between the knee and the ankle at the front of the leg).

Arthritis: Requires whole body treatment; also channel Reiki locally and apply positions 13 and 17.

Arthrosis: Treat locally and with positions 13, 14, 17.

Asthma: Apply positions 1, 4, 9 and 10.

Backache: Give local treatment and apply positions 1, 11, 12, 15 and 17.

Bed-wetting: Apply positions 5, 8, 10, 11 and 13. Parents or attendants should also be treated with Reiki for some time.

Bilious Complaints: Work with positions 1, 6, 12, 15 and 17; specific Reiki work on the third chakra is to be recommended in the case of chronic disorders.

Bladder: Use positions 4, 10, 11, 14 and 16; for chronic complaints, specific Reiki work on the second chakra is additionally recommended.

Bleeding: Channel in Reiki at the wound; if there is severe loss of blood, do positions 1, 5, 7, 13 and 17. Reiki does not make first aid superfluous in the case of bleeding.

Blood Pressure: In the case of high blood pressure, apply positions 5, 6 and 17; in the case of low blood pressure use positions 11, 12, 14 and 17.

Breathing Difficulties: Apply positions 4, 9 and 17.

Bronchial system: Do positions 1, 9, and 11, and place your hands below the chest on the ribs.

Burns: Give local treatment, but do not touch the burns! In serious cases also give regular whole body treatment, especially with positions 1, 6, 9, 13, 14 and 17.

Cancer (also see Detoxification): Carry out whole body treatment regularly and channel Reiki to the afflicted areas if known. Work a lot with positions 6 and 8, keep position 9 for about 15 to 20 minutes, do specific Reiki work on the fourth chakra and balance out the chakras via the fourth chakra. In the case of extreme weakness apply positions 14 and 17, and do chakra balancing at the first and sixth chakras. In the case of tongue cancer also channel Reiki into the body from the feet. In the case of breast cancer and cancer of the urogenital system, do additional intensive work with positions 10, 14 and 16 and supplement with specific Reiki work on the second chakra.

Cancerous Ulcers: Channel Reiki energy into the soles of the feet and carry out local treatment at regular intervals but only for a few minutes.

Cardiac Enlargement: Channel in Reiki at the area above the nipples and work with positions 2 and 3.

Cardiac Infarction: Channel Reiki into the upper and lower abdomen and do position 13.

Caries: Apply positions 1, 6, 10, 14, 15 and 17 and do specific work on the first chakra.

Chemotherapy (for cancer): Treat before and a few hours after receiving treatment. If regular medication is taken, only do specific Reiki work with positions 6, 7, 9, 10 and 13. If medication is only taken once, do several whole body treatments afterwards and the same positions as above.

Childbirth: Whole body treatment beforehand and apply positions 8, 10, 13 and 14. Reiki helps the expectant mother to relax and facilitates the opening of the pelvis. Therefore the birth is less painful, with the child more easily finding an ideal position.

Chilliness: Work with positions 1, 8, 13, 14 and 17. If there is frequent shivering for no external reason (hypothermia), supply the second chakra with Reiki.

Circulation: Do positions 1, 5, 6 and 8, channel Reiki energy into the tops of the shoulders, above the chest, a handsbreadth below the armpits and into the crotch from the inside of the thighs and place hands to the right and left of the top of the head.

Colds (also see Inflammation): Do positions 1, 5 and 9.

Constipation (also see Digestive Complaints): Place one hand below the navel and the other on the nape of the neck.

Cough (also see Inflammation): Channel in Reiki at the upper back and do positions 1, 5, and 9.

Cramps: Treat locally (but consult a physician if there is a tendency to cramps); also apply positions 1, 6, 12, 13, 15 and 17 and do specific work on the sixth chakra (Third Eye).

Deafness: Treat with positions 3, 5, and 9 and in serious cases do specific Reiki work on the fifth chakra.

Depression: Carry out whole body treatment and do positions 1, 4, 10 and 17.

Detoxification: Carry out regular whole body treatment on consecutive days until there is the first sign of a healing reaction (such as darker urine with a different smell, perspiration, bowel movement, skin reactions). The patient should drink a lot of spring or mineral water, take showers and rest as much as possible. Also apply positions 1, 5 to 10, 13, 14 and 17. Treatment of the central shoulder region to the right and left of the spine is also very effective. In the case of weakened kidney and/or liver function the patient should only be treated in consultation with a physician or a practitioner of natural therapeutics.

Diabetes: Work with the special diabetes position (at the elbow) and apply positions 1, 7, 9 and 17.

Diarrhoea: Apply positions 6, 7, 8, 10 and 13.

Digestive Complaints: Apply positions 4, 6, 8, 10, 11, 12, 14 and 16.

Dizziness: Treat with positions 3, 6, 14 and 17 and place the hands crossways over the top of the head.

Duodenal Ulcer: Treat locally and apply positions 1, 6, 8 and 10 (also see Inflammation).

Dyspnea: Apply positions 4, 8 and 17 and also treat the shoulder region.

Ear Complaints and Conditions: Apply positions 1, 5, and 17 and channel Reiki into the inside of the feet, particularly in the area between the big toe and the arch of the foot.

Eczema (also see Rash): Treat the chest and upper back.

Electric Shock: As a first aid measure, apply Reiki to the wrists and call a physician immediately (also see Heart in general and Shock).

Emphysema: Carry out whole body treatment; channel Reiki into the collar bone, chest and back and apply positions 5 and 17.

Epileptic Fits: Work with positions 4, 5, 8 and allow Reiki to flow into the wrists and the section of the spine between the shoulder blades, but only before or after a seizure.

Exhaustion: Carry out whole body treatment and do positions 17, 14, 13 and 8. (in this order).

Eye Complaints: Do positions 1, 2, 5, 10 and 17 and channel Reiki energy into the big toes and/or the thumb.

Fasting: Work with positions 5, 8, 10, 12, 14 and 17.

Fatigue: Carry out chakra balancing and apply positions 1, 2, 10, 14 and 17.

Fear: Do positions 8, 13, 14, and 17; in extreme cases you can also place your hands on the top of the head if you want to reduce fear of physical closeness and help your client to open up or close himself off in a healthy manner, treat the elbows (inside and outside).

Fever: Apply positions 1, 3, 5, 7 and 9 and complement with whole body treatment and positions 14 and 17 in the case of a high or prolonged temperature. The patient will often react with an increase in temperature which, however, soon subsides(also see Inflammation).

Flatulence: Do positions 4, 6, 7 and 8 and channel Reiki into the ankles and heels.

Fractures: After the bones have been set, treat locally for long periods on a frequent basis and also work with positions 1, 6, 14, 17.

Frigidity: Employ positions 1, 8 and 14 and supplement with Reiki specifically applied to the second and fifth chakras. Both partners should also be given regular whole body treatment; the same applies to chakra work. The causes of sexual problems affecting a partnership generally lie with both partners.

Gastric disorders: Apply positions 6 and 8 and if chronic, complement with specific Reiki work on the sixth chakra and also apply position 12.

Gingivitis: Treat locally (also see Inflammation and Caries).

Gland complaints: Apply positions 1, 4, 10, 12, 14 and 16.

Glaucoma: Allow Reiki to act in the region of the eyes and work with positions 1 and 5; do specific Reiki work on the second and sixth chakras and also treat the complete length of the big toes.

Goiter: Channel Reiki two handbreadths above the ankles and work with positions 5, 9, 10 and 14.

Gout: Channel in Reiki at the affected spots and apply positions 8, 12 and 13.

Hair loss: Apply Reiki locally as well as positions 10, 13 and 16.

Hangover (due to alcohol or drug abuse): Apply Reiki a handsbreadth above the ankles and treat the whole of the big toes.(Also see Detoxification, Headache, Nausea and Indigestion).

Hay fever (also see Allergy): Provide regular treatment using positions 1, 4, 10, 12, 13 and 16.

Headache: Work with positions 1, 4, 11, 12, and 17. (You do not have to use all at once; apply whatever seems most effective.)

Heart Attack: Apply Reiki treatment to the upper and lower abdomen (but in no circumstances directly to the heart) along with positions 6, 8, 11 and 13. This is only to be used as an emergency measure until the physician arrives.

Heart Trouble, general: Treat the second and fourth chakra for all kinds of heart trouble. The client must also consult a physician or a practitioner of natural therapeutics.

Heartburn: Apply positions 8 and 4.

Haemorrhoids: Provide Reiki locally and also positions 6, 8, 11, 12, 14, 16 and 17.

Hepatitis (inflammation of the liver): Use the same treatments as described under Inflammation and Liver; also do specific work on the first and third chakras and apply position 12.

Hiccups: The person with hiccups raises his arms in the air and the person treating him places one hand on the solar plexus and the other above it; in the case of frequent recurrence, additional work should be carried out with position 4.

Hoarseness: Local treatment; in the case of frequent hoarseness, do specific Reiki work on the fifth chakra.

Hot Flushes: Apply positions 8 and 10 and do chakra balancing on the second and third chakra.

Hyperactivity: Give regular whole body treatment and channel Reiki in at the top of the head; apply positions 2, 3, 6 and 8 and do specific work on the fifth chakra.

Hypoglycaemia: Work with positions 6 and 13 and the special diabetes position.

Hysteria: (also see Panic): Channel Reiki in at both the wrists and crossways across the top of the head and then massage the hands vigorously for a few minutes; apply positions 8, 12 and 17.

Imbalance: Apply position 3 and 6 and place both hands on the top of the head.

Impotence: Work with positions 1, 8, 10, 12 and 14 and in serious cases do specific Reiki work on the second and fifth chakras. It is best to include both partners in the treatment as sexual problems affecting partnerships almost generally lie with both partners.

Inflammation: Channel Reiki locally, that is at the focus of the inflammation and also do positions 7, 9, 10, 14, and 17. For chronic/severe inflammation, also consider positions 6 and 13 and treat lymph nodes in those areas. Specific Reiki work on the sixth chakra (Third Eye) is also recommended. Chakra balancing should be carried out, especially on the first and sixth chakras, and an oracle should be consulted to determine whether a decision has been put off; this is generally the cause of all inflammation. Precious stone work can also be performed with amethyst and rock crystal.

Influenza: Whole body treatment (also see "Inflammation" and "Fever").

Injuries: Treat locally, but do not touch. (also see Shock and Accident)

Insomnia: Apply positions 1, 2, 8 and 10 and channel Reiki into the collarbone; in the case of frequent insomnia do specific work on the third chakra.

Knee Complaints: Work with positions 15 and 17 and the special sciatica position; put both your hands around the knee so it is able to absorb Reiki from all sides. If chronic, also work on the third and sixth chakra.

Kidney: Apply positions 1, 10, 13, 14 and 16 and do Reiki work on the second chakra in the case of chronic complaints.

Large Intestine, Complaints of: Do positions 4, 6, 7, 8, 10 and 14 and also treat the inside of the lower leg from the knee to the ankle.

Laryngeal Complaints: Work with position 5 and treat the whole of the big toe. If chronic, also work on the fifth chakra.

Legs: Carry out specific Reiki work on the Third Eye along with positions 1, 14, 15, 16, 17 and the special sciatica position.

Leukaemia: Regular whole body treatment and intensive work with positions 6, 8, 10, 14, 16 and 17; also perform specific Reiki work on the first and second chakras.

Liver Complaints: Apply positions 6, 8 and 12.

Medication (side effects and effects of drugs): No prolonged whole body treatment should be given during the administration of medication which has to remain in the body at constant levels (i.e. anticoagulants, cardiac stimulants or chemotherapeutic drugs) but you may work with positions 5, 6, 13, 14 and 17 (also see Detoxification"). Treat organic damage caused by drugs locally and give Reiki whole body treatment.

Memory Problems: In the case of poor memory or loss of memory, place hands crossways over the top of the head.

Meningitis (also see Inflammation): Treat the big toes and the thumbs with Reiki and do positions 1 to 4.

Menstrual Complaints: Apply positions 6, 8, 10, 12, 14, 16 and 17 and carry out specific Reiki work on the second chakra. Local treatment can be accompanied by strong cramps/pain caused by the fear of physical touch and movement; in this case it is better to apply positions 16 and 17.

Metabolic Diseases: Whole body treatment is absolutely necessary! Additionally apply positions 1, 5, 8, 14 and 17.

Migraine (also see Headache): Apply positions 10, 14 and 16.

Mouth Complaints and Conditions: Give local treatment and apply position 1; also infuse Reiki at the big toes and thumbs.

Mucous Catarrh: Treat with positions 1, 6, 8, 12, 14 and 17.

Multiple Sclerosis (also see Inflammation): Use the special cranium position and do specific Reiki work on the sixth chakra. If two Reiki initiates are available for the treatment, one of them places his hands on the head and the other on the soles of the feet. Whole body treatment and local treatment of the affected areas is also to be recommended. Apply positions 1, 4, and 8 and treat the area between the shoulders.

Nausea: Apply positions 6 and 8 and in the case of car sickness, work with positions 3 and 6; place hands on the top of the head.

Neck Pains: Channel in Reiki energy to the area of pain and to the main joint of the big toes and work with positions 8 and 10.

Nervous Heart Trouble: Treat both sides of the body a handsbreadth below the armpits and use positions 2, 3, 9, 11 and 13.

Nervous Breakdown: Apply positions 1, 4, 8, 10, 11, 12, 14 and 17 and place hands crossways over the top of the head.

Nervousness: Channel in Reiki at the base of the thumb, at the base of the big toes on the top of the foot and at the cranium (putting both hands across the head) and work with positions 1, 5 and 8.

Neuralgia: Treat locally and via the reflex zones and also use positions 1 and 17 and, very intensively, position 16.

Neurosis: Do chakra balancing frequently and regularly. Find out which chakra/organ is causing the disorder and carry out specific Reiki work in that area; also apply positions 5, 8, 12 and 17. Whole body treatment is also recommended at weekly intervals.

Nightmares: Carry out positions 2, 4, 8 and 10.'

Nose Complaints and Conditions: Give local treatment and apply positions 1, 6 and 9; also carry out specific Reiki work on the sixth chakra. In the case of sinus problems, also work with positions 10, 12, 14 and 16 and complement with specific Reiki work on the second chakra.

Nosebleeds: Treat locally and apply positions 4, 5, 8, 11 and 12.

Numbness: Place the hands between the spine and the lower ends of the shoulder blades.

Nymphomania: Apply positions 1, 5, 10 and 16 and carry out specific Reiki work on the second and fifth chakras.

Operations: Apply whole body treatment beforehand along with positions 8 and 9 and whole body treatment afterwards as a recuperative measure. Channel Reiki into the scars and also work with positions 6, 8, 12-14 and 17.

Pain: Treat locally and apply positions 11 and 12. Bone pains: Place one hand above and one hand below the main cervical vertebra at the nape of the neck. Hip and leg pains: Channel in Reiki along the whole back and the outside of the hips. Arm pains: Apply positions 11 and 12 and channel in Reiki on the top of the shoulders and arms. Leg pains: apply positions 13 and 14 and treat the outside of the hips.

Panic (stage fever): Channel Reiki in at the wrists and the outside of the knees; apply positions 4, 8, 12 and 13.

Perspiration: Apply positions 10, 13, 15, 16 and 17 and also channel Reiki into the palms two finger breadths away from the base of the thumb.

Pleurisy: Treat locally and channel Reiki below the armpits; apply position 1 (also see Inflammation).

Pneumonia (also see Inflammation): Medical treatment is an absolute necessity in this case. As a supportive measure, simultaneously channel in Reiki at the chest and from the top of the back and also treat the wrists and the base of the thumb with Reiki (the sessions should take place daily and never be shorter than ten minutes).

Poisoning: Call a physician immediately! (also see Detoxification)

Postural Anomalies: Give the fifth chakra specific Reiki treatment and treat the chakra where the postural anomaly is most evident; also treat the inside of the feet from the big toe to the heel.

Rash: Apply whole body treatment and positions 5, 6, 10, 12 and 13; also carry out specific Reiki work on the sixth chakra (Third Eye)

Rheumatism: Apply whole body treatment and positions 8, 10, 13 and 15.

Scars: Treat locally and apply positions 5, 8 and 9.

Scheuermann's disease: Apply whole body treatment and channel Reiki into the back in particular; apply positions 10, 14 and 17 and do specific Reiki work on the first chakra.

Sciatica: Apply the special sciatica position.

Shock: As a first aid measure, apply positions 8 and 13 and then the sides of the shoulders. Follow up later with whole body treatment and in particular apply positions 1, 4, 8, 10, 12, 14 and 17.

Skin Complaints and Conditions: Treat locally and perform specific Reiki work on the second chakra (also see Detoxification).

Sluggishness: Carry out whole body treatment and apply positions 6, 10, 14 and 17 in particular; also channel Reiki to the front of the legs a handsbreadth below the knees.

Smoking, Giving Up: Do specific Reiki work on the sixth and first chakras and also apply positions 1, 4, 5, 6, 8, 10, 13 and 17.

Sore throat: Treat locally and also the whole of the big toes.

Splenic Complaints: Apply position 8 and give specific Reiki treatment to the second chakra.

Sprains: Immediately treat locally for about 15 to 20 minutes; repeat two or three times a day for a few days. A physician is to be consulted to exclude the possibility of joint damage.

Stab Wounds: Treat locally and in the case of shock apply positions 8 and 13 and channel Reiki into the tops of the shoulders.

Stammering: Channel Reiki below the collarbone to the left and right and also apply position 5.

Stroke: Channel Reiki into the side of the head opposite the part of the body affected by the stroke (that is, the right side of the head for the left side of the body, and vice versa). Call a physician immediately.

Tachycardia: Treat the wrists with Reiki and apply positions 5, 8 and 17.

Teeth: Have their own reflex zones which may be treated in the case of toothache (or caries) with Reiki. These reflex zones are as follows: the big toes for the incisors; the second toes for the canines; the middle toes for the premolars; the fourth toes for the molars and the small toes for the wisdom teeth. Furthermore each tooth is energetically connected with some organ or region of the body, and therefore the latter should also be treated with Reiki regularly in the case of diseases of the teeth. If all the teeth are carious, as a rule this will have to do with a deep-seated metabolic disease. To facilitate treatment, there now follows a list of the teeth and the organs and regions of the body that are associated with an energetic level.

Incisors: Kidney and bladder meridian, urogenital system, the ears, nasal and frontal sinuses, adenoids, coccyx, root chakra.

Canines: Liver and gall bladder meridian, the eyes, hips, thoracic spine, the pituitary gland, the knees, palatine tonsils.

Anterior premolars (upper): Lung and large intestine meridian, nose, nasal sinuses, bronchial tubes, hands, shoulders, knees, upper sections of the spine, the pituitary and thymus glands.

Anterior premolars (lower right and left): Larynx, mammary glands, pharynx, gonads, lymph vessels, knees, jaw and maxillary sinuses.

Anterior premolars (lower right): Pancreas and stomach meridian.

Anterior premolars (lower left): Spleen and stomach meridian.

Molars (upper right and left): Jaw and maxillary sinuses, knees, thyroid gland, parathyroid, mammary glands.

Molars (upper right): Pancreas and stomach meridian.

Molars (upper left): Spleen and stomach meridian.

Molars (lower right and left): Lung and large intestine meridian, arteries and veins, nose, nasal sinuses, bronchial tubes.

Wisdom teeth (upper right and left): Heart and small intestine meridian, middle ear, shoulders, elbow.

Wisdom teeth (upper right): Central nervous system, duodenum.

Wisdom teeth (upper left): Lower section of the small intestine, jejunum.

Wisdom teeth (lower right and left): Heart and small intestine meridian, shoulders, elbows, middle ear.

Wisdom teeth (lower right): Lower section of the small intestine; **wisdom teeth (lower left)**: Jejunum. There is also an energetic connection between the teeth and the thoracic vertebrae.

Teething: Apply positions 1, 14, and 17 and lay a hand above the mouth or on the cheek.

Tenosynovitis: Treat locally; in the case of frequent occurrence also apply positions 1 and 5 and treat the sixth chakra.

Tension: Treat locally and apply positions 1, 8, 12 and 13; supplement with Reiki work on the sixth chakra for chronic tension.

Thyroid gland: Apply positions 1, 5, 9 and 12; and carry out specific Reiki work on the fifth chakra.

Tonsillitis (also see Inflammation): Work with positions 1, 3, 5, 9 and 13.

Toothache: Treat locally (also see Caries and Teeth).

Ulcers and Boils: Apply Reiki locally (in the case of boils etc. do not touch the skin); in the case of a stomach ulcer, also treat the outside of the upper arms.

Ulcer of the Breast: Give frequent whole body treatment and also apply positions 10, 14 and 17. Specific work on the second and fourth chakras is also important.

Unconsciousness: Channel Reiki into the upper side of the big toes and do positions 5, 8, 14 and 17.

Venereal Diseases: Must be notified to the authorities and may only be treated by physicians; supporting treatment can be provided in the form of specific Reiki work on the first, second and sixth chakras (also see Inflammation).

Weakness: Treat the lower abdomen, the sacrum, the kidneys and the soles of the feet.

Weight, Problems: Apply positions 1, 5, 8, 10, 12, 14 and 16 and do specific Reiki work on the second and fifth chakras.

Whiplash Injury (also see Shock): Apply positions 4, 11, 14 and 17 and place one hand above and the other below the main cervical vertebra at the nape of the neck.

Directions for the Use of the Pendulum Dowsing Tables

The pendulum dowsing tables are meant to help you find the most effective methods of treatment for each respective situation and, if you wish, to probe deeper into the causes. As I have already pointed out, such tools become more and more dispensable with time, which is perfectly desirable. Until then, pendulum dowsing and oracle work may provide a great deal of good advice on dealing with Reiki. Since it is impossible to provide tables on everything, I have provided some of the tables with typical alternatives and left the others free for your own use. You may fill them out according to your own ideas, and create your own system of analysis. In all the tables I have filled out you'll find a section marked "error". This is important as this is where the pendulum will move if the pertinent reason is not included in the table or you are unable to gain meaningful results with it at the moment. You can gain more information on the obstacle by using the Error Table. If you want to work with the pendulum on a matter which is very important for you, you should ask the pendulum a few times whether the result is really true and, if there's any doubt, consult a pendulum dowser who is not emotionally involved in the matter. Oracle work with the "I Ching", tarot cards or runes is to be recommended in this instance to exclude errors as far as possible. If you have never worked seriously with a pendulum before, or only have little experience, attend a good seminar, do some reading on the subject or practice for some time on simple problems before tackling important ones, otherwise the whole business can go very wrong.

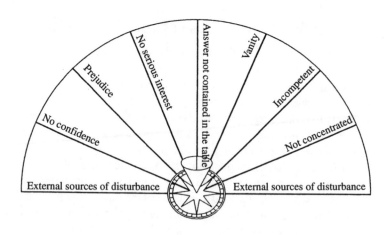

Error table

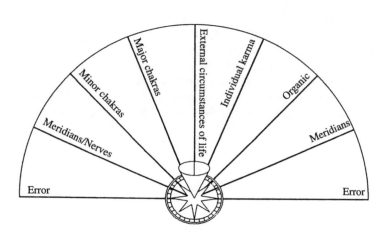

Causes

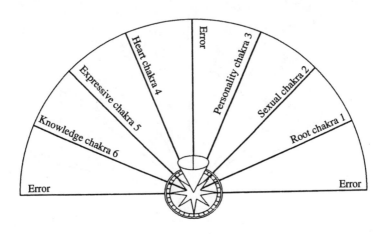

The six major chakras

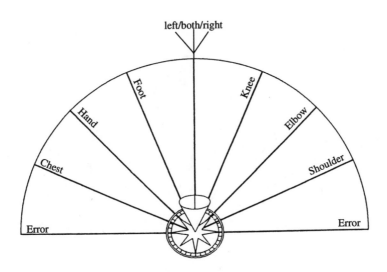

Minor chakras

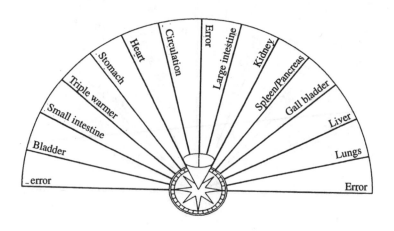

The 12 meridians

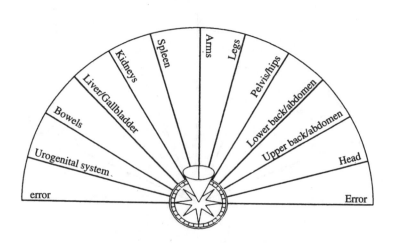

Organs and bodily zones

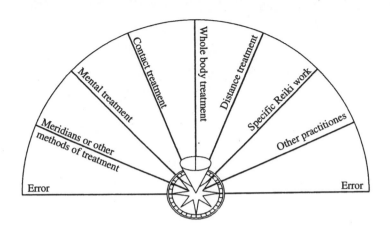

Treatment

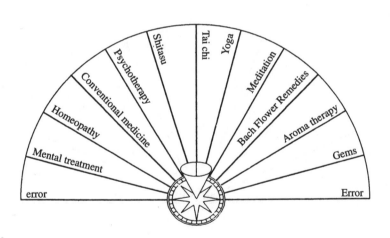

Additional aids

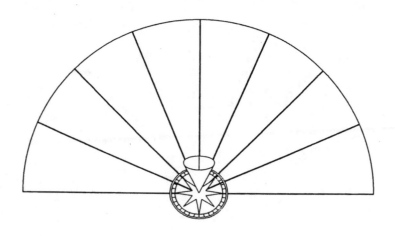

Pendulum tables to label yourself

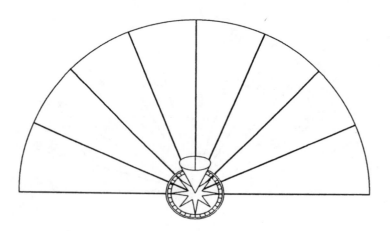

Cleaning Jewelry on the Energy Level

Forget anything that you've ever heard to the contrary, and never clean your jewelry with salt! This is more harmful than useful and may even totally destroy certain gems.

Useful methods of cleaning:
- Get hold of some dry, clean silica and leave it in the sun for a few days. The sun will clean it on an energy level and charge it with positive energy. Now bury your jewelry in the sand for a day, and then rinse it briefly in cold water.
- Hold the jewelry under cold, running water for a few minutes. The colder the water the better as cold water draws the energy from the gems.
- Put your jewelry in a sunny spot for a few days and rinse it in cold water afterwards.
- If you have no other way of cleaning your jewelry, you can clean it with Reiki energy and visualization. Take it into your hands and imagine that you are holding it in a stream of cool mountain water. With your inner eye, watch how dark clouds of disharmonious energy are washed out of the gems. Continue until there is no longer any discoloration of the water. Your jewelry will then be clean.
- Before applying any of the described methods, ensure that your aura is free from disturbing energy, at least at your hands and forearms.
- The basic rule is; whatever jewelry you wear, you should clean it every day you wear it, particularly if you come into contact with lots of people or have to face a lot of stressful situations.

Addresses and List of Supply Sources

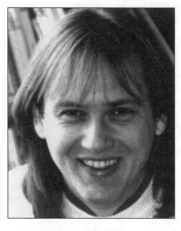

If you would like to contact **Walter Lübeck** and **The Reiki Do Institute**, please write to:

✉

Windpferd Verlag
"The Complete Reiki Handbook"
Friesenrieder Strasse 45
87648 Aitrang
Germany

Sources for fragrances, flower remedies, herbs, gemstones and music cassettes:

Wholesale (contact with your business name and resale number or practitioner licence):

Lotus Light
P.O.Box 1008 RH
Silver Lake, WI 53170
☎   262 889 8501
Fax   262 889 8591

Retail / Mail Order:
International
33719 116th St. Box RH
Twin Lakes, WI 53181
800/643-4221
www.internatural.com

More from the Shangri-La series:

Dr. Paula Horan
Empowerment through Reiki
The path to personal and global transformation—a handbook
192 pages, US $ 14,95
ISBN 0-941524-84-1

Shalila Sharamon and Bodo J. Baginski
The Chakra-Handbook
From basic understanding to practical application. A comprehensive guide to harmonising the energy centers
192 pages, US $ 14,95
ISBN 0-941524-85-X

Marianne Uhl
Chakra Energy Massage
Spiritual evolution into the subconscious through activation of the energy points of the feet
128 pages, US $ 9,95
ISBN 0-941524-83-3

Dr. Paula Horan
Brigitte Ziegler MA.
Dissolving Co-dependency
Powerful insights from the Core-Empowerment-Training
106 pages, US $ 9,95
ISBN 0-941524-86-8